Modern Nutrition for Busy Families
By Cindy Silver, MS, RDN, LDN
and Andrea Collare Everhart

ISBN# 978-1984371461

Disclaimer: Always consult with your doctor or your kids' doctor about health and nutrition. The information in this book is not intended to replace the advice of a doctor, but only to supplement it.

Less Sugary Homemade Lemonade from Cover Photo
Kids can help by squeezing the lemons, measuring the ingredients and stirring, with supervision.

Makes 3-4 servings

2 large, juicy	Lemons, or 3 small lemons
2 cups	Water
2 level tablespoons	Sugar

1. Cut lemons in half, squeeze juice into small pitcher and discard seeds.
2. Add water and sugar.
3. Stir well to dissolve all sugar.
4. Taste and add 1 level teaspoon sugar if needed.

I dedicate this book to my son, Jay, for helping me tweak my skills at cooking nutritiously in a way that pleases kids. I also dedicate this book to my mom, all busy moms, and all my nutrition clients. You are a huge inspiration to me.
Cindy

To my girls, who lament often that they have to eat the healthiest packed lunches in the school, I dedicate this book. With some of these great tips from Cindy, I now have hope that we can encourage everyone to incorporate nutrition into their lives and make it a little more fun for each of them!

Andrea

Contents

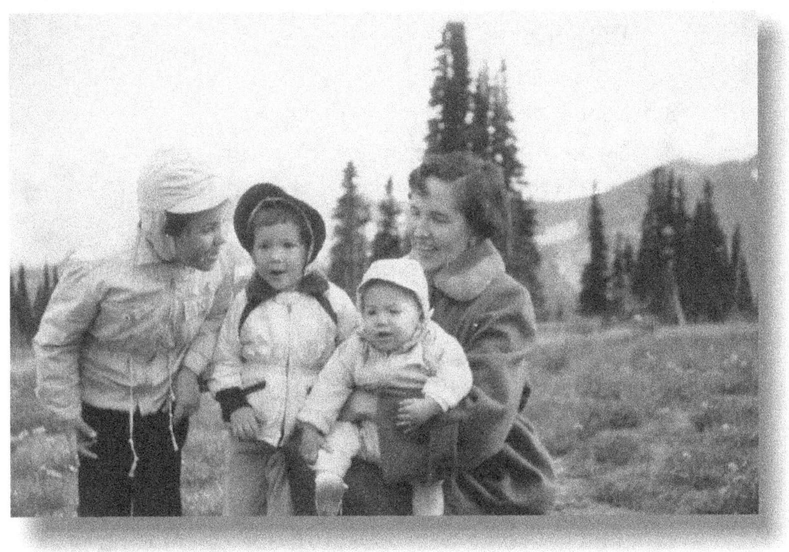

What's Modern Nutrition?

Modern nutrition makes it possible for modern families to thrive, day-after-day. It is simple foods made into plans for tasty and nutritious meals. It is go-to snacks that keep energy levels high - morning, noon, and night. It is easy recipes with quality nutrition, even for special occasion meals. Modern nutrition helps you deal with a busy schedule and fit in foods with great flavors, textures, and nutrients. When everyone in the house is hungry, time is tight and you want more than ever to resist another take-out order, modern nutrition saves the day. Come to this handy resource for an easy weeknight meal plan, a way to cook vegetables so they will be eaten, a creative themed dinner, fun snacks, a party plan, and more. Remember that small victories add up to winning the war of feeding your family well.

10 Modern Cooking Rules

1. Tell yourself, "I can do this!"
2. Embrace easy.
3. Repeat meals when you must.
4. Never apologize for how dinner turns out.
5. Keep a go-to dinner always stocked in your pantry or freezer – just in case.
6. Buy cooked chicken or grab pre-made sandwiches or a salad bar meal at the grocery store when you are in a time crunch.
7. Cook in a big batch on Saturday or Sunday and use these meals for your busiest weeknights. See *5 Slow Cooker Recipes* (page 91) for batch recipe ideas.
8. Get some input on meal ideas from your family and then get some help cooking it and cleaning up.
9. Write down your dinner plan then make a grocery list to stay organized.
10. Find the fun in cooking!

Safety Tips for Young Kids

Keep these in mind, especially when preparing and serving food to **kids under five years old:**

- Hot dogs and sausages – cut into very small, irregular pieces
- Carrots – finely shred or cook to soft
- Apples – cut into very small pieces or cook to soft
- Celery – cut into very small pieces or cook to soft
- Grapes and Cherries – cut in halves or fourths
- Nut Butter – spread in a thin layer on cracker or bread
- Avoid nuts, marshmallows, popcorn, pretzels, cheese cubes, melon cubes and round and/or hard candies
- Offer water to sip between mouthfuls

- Make sure kids are seated while eating
- Be cautious and observant when using toothpicks

♥ **Bright Idea!** *To keep a safe and healthy kitchen, learn and use food safety strategies every single day. For helpful details, check out the Partnership for Food Safety Education (www.fightbac.org) online.*

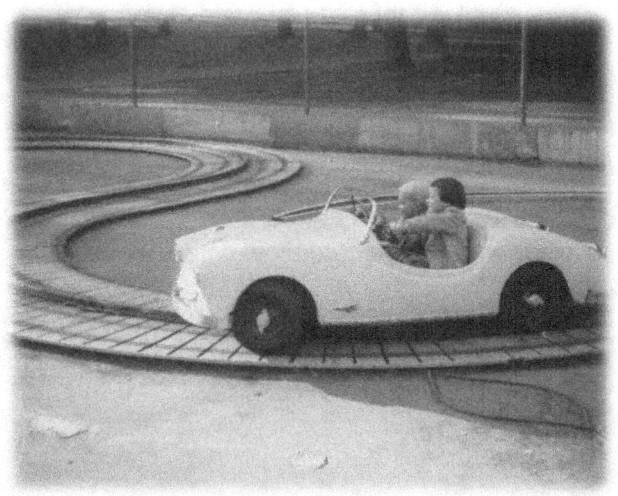

Super Speedy Meal Tips

Life moves at a fast pace and it's a challenge to keep-up with eating well. We get it. Here are 15 nutritious & super speedy meal options to get you going on your busiest days. Try a few at a time.

Note: If you are doing an in-the-car meal, then look for the ones with *

Breakfast

- Banana & Nut Butter Wrap* – Smear peanut/almond/soy nut butter onto a whole wheat tortilla and then wrap it around a peeled banana.
- Cheese & Greens Pocket* – Stuff sliced cheese and lettuce/spinach/arugula greens into a whole grain pocket bread. Drizzle with vinaigrette dressing.
- Jazzed Up Yogurt – Scoop out vanilla yogurt into a cereal bowl, then add mixed nuts, raisins, sunflower or pumpkin seeds.

- Savory Oatmeal with an Egg on Top – At the same time, and in different pans, cook oatmeal and fry an egg in extra virgin olive oil. Season the cooked oatmeal with 1 teaspoon soy, gochujang, or barbecue sauce. Put the cooked egg on top.
- Hummus & Avocado Toast – Make whole grain toast. Spread on hummus. Top with avocado slices.

Lunch

- Healthier Ramen Noodles – Cook ramen noodles with ½ the spice packet. Top it off with canned tuna or canned chicken, grape tomatoes and soybeans (edamame.)
- Turkey & Light Cream Cheese Wrap* – Smear light cream cheese on a whole grain pita wrap, then add sliced turkey and sprinkle with dried cranberries.
- Tuna or Chicken Salad Plate – Cover a plate with spinach or lettuce, then add a scoop of tuna salad or chicken salad. Finish with almonds and diced apples on top.
- Cottage Cheese & Fruit – Scoop out 1% cottage cheese into a cereal bowl, then add cut up pineapple, peaches, and/or berries. Eat with a couple of grainy crackers for crunch.
- Butter and Fruit Sandwich* – Choose a whole grain bread, wrap, pita, or cracker. Smear on peanut butter, almond butter, or sunflower butter. Add sliced fruit such as apple, pear, melon, plum, or grapes.

Dinner

- Slow Cooker Option – Check our Slow Cooker Recipes on pages 91-95. Come home to a homemade dinner.
- Chili over Rice – Make your own or purchase canned chili and serve over brown rice.
- Grilled Cheese with a Mediterranean Twist – Spread your whole grain bread with basil pesto, add a sliced

tomato and a slice of Provolone cheese. Cook as usual for grilled cheese. Optional: Add arugula, too.

- Southwestern Omelet – Use 2 eggs to make a simple omelet, then top with canned black beans, prepared salsa and chopped fresh cilantro.
- Roasted Chunks of Sweet Potato, Red Onion and Cauliflower with Hummus to Dip – Buy pre-cut sweet potatoes and cauliflower florets. Cut red onion into chunks. Cook according to our recipe for Roasted Vegetables on page 102.

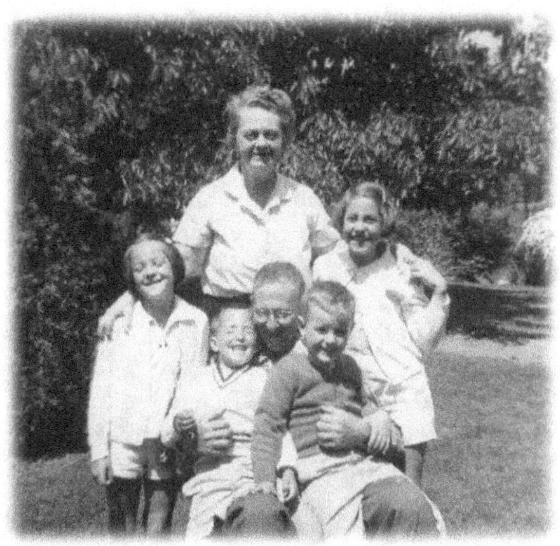

Modern Weeknight Meals

This section is to help you with ideas. As you try our 15 meals, practice these 5 easy steps as a way to get more organized, comfortable and confident in the kitchen.

5 Steps to Meal Planning and Cooking Success

1. Pick out a meal to make and read through the lead recipe slowly.
2. Read over the shopping list, taking items off the shopping list that you already have on-hand.
3. Grocery shop for the meal with the handy list provided.
4. Get organized to cook and/or assemble the meal.
5. Store any leftovers and use them up within 2-3 days.

♥ **Bright Idea!** *A well-lit, clean and uncluttered kitchen is a nice place to be. So, be sure to pick up and get organized for a great cooking experience!*

Meal 1: Meatball Sub Sandwich

Meatball Sub with Red Marinara Sauce & Melted Cheese
Peas
Apple Slices with Cinnamon Sprinkled on Top
1% Milk or Water

Meatball Recipe (6 servings):

1. Preheat oven to 400 degrees.
2. Mix together **1 pound lean ground beef** or turkey breast + pinch of **salt** + pinch of **ground black pepper** + ½ teaspoon of **garlic powder** + ½ teaspoon of **onion powder** + ½ **cup bread crumbs** or **oatmea**l.
3. Add **1 large egg** and ½ **cup low fat or nonfat milk**.
4. Make little meatballs about 1-1/2 inch balls and place onto a flat sheet pan 1 inch apart.
5. Bake at 400 degrees for 15 minutes. Cool.
6. Enjoy right away or freeze for later.

Note: To assemble the meatball sub, place 3 cooked meatballs into the **sub roll** and top with warmed-up **red Marinara sauce** and **Mozzarella cheese**. The cheese will melt on top, becoming soft, stretchy and fun.

Check out our handy grocery list on the next page to save you some time. Snap a picture of it with your Smart Phone and bring it with you on your shopping trip!

<u>Meal 1 Grocery List:</u>

- ☐ Frozen peas
- ☐ Fresh apples
- ☐ Ground cinnamon
- ☐ 1% Milk

For Meatball Sub Recipe

- ☐ 1 pound lean ground beef or turkey breast
- ☐ Salt and black pepper
- ☐ Garlic powder
- ☐ Onion powder
- ☐ Bread crumbs or plain oatmeal
- ☐ Egg
- ☐ Low fat or nonfat milk
- ☐ Submarine rolls, 6 inches long (half a sub is typically enough for young kids)
- ☐ Mozzarella cheese, shredded (or buy a chunk of cheese and grate it yourself)

NOTES:

____

____

____

____

____

____

____

____

Meal 2: Grilled Cheese & Tuna

Grilled Cheese & Canned Tuna
Baby Carrots & Greek Yogurt Dip
Strawberry & Orange Smoothie

Strawberry & Orange Smoothie Recipe (3 servings):

1. Put the following into your blender: **1 cup frozen unsweetened strawberries,** partly thawed with their juice + **1 cup orange juice + ¾ cup lemon yogurt + ¼ cup plain yogurt**.
2. Blend on high for 1 minute.

Check out our handy grocery list on the next page to save you some time. Snap a picture of it with your Smart Phone and bring it with you on your shopping trip!

<u>Meal 2 Grocery List:</u>

- ☐ Whole grain wheat or white wheat bread
- ☐ Cheese
- ☐ Canned tuna
- ☐ Baby carrots
- ☐ Greek yogurt dip (or make your own using plain Greek style yogurt)

For Smoothie Recipe

- ☐ Frozen unsweetened strawberries
- ☐ Orange juice
- ☐ Lemon yogurt
- ☐ Plain yogurt

NOTES:

____

____

____

____

____

____

____

____

____

Meal 3: Eggs with Waffles

Scrambled Eggs
Frozen Toaster Waffles, whole grain
Canned Peaches with cottage cheese
1% Milk or Water

Easy Scrambled Eggs Recipe (2 servings):

1. Crack **3-4 eggs** into a small bowl, add **1 tablespoon water** and scramble them with a fork or whisk.
2. Heat a medium skillet/pan to medium heat on the stovetop, about 3-4 minutes.
3. Add **½ tablespoon butter or oil**.
4. Pour the eggs into the pan and allow them to cook gradually while you stir with a fork or wooden spoon.
5. Season lightly with **salt** and **pepper**.
6. Remove from pan when eggs are cooked, about 4-6 minutes.

Check out our handy grocery list on the next page to save you some time. Snap a picture of it with your Smart Phone and bring it with you on your shopping trip!

<u>Meal 3 Grocery List:</u>
- ☐ Frozen whole grain toaster waffles
- ☐ Canned peaches, in their own juice
- ☐ 1% Cottage cheese (optional)
- ☐ 1% Milk

For Scrambled Eggs Recipe
- ☐ Fresh eggs
- ☐ Butter or olive/canola oil
- ☐ Salt and pepper

NOTES:

____

____

____

____

____

____

____

____

____

Meal 4: Quick Chicken Noodle Soup with Half Sandwich

Quick Chicken Noodle Soup
Half Peanut Butter & Raisin Sandwich, whole grain or white
wheat bread
(or switch the raisins to banana slices)
Cucumber Slices & Hummus
1% Milk or Water

Quick Chicken Noodle Soup Recipe (4 bowls of soup):

1. Get out a medium pot with a lid & heat to medium-high, then add **1 tablespoon olive or canola oil.**
2. Lightly sauté **½ cup** each in the heated pot: cut-up **celery, carrots, onion** and **fresh parsley**.
3. Stir the vegetables for 3-4 minutes until slightly soft.
4. Add **1 quart (32 fluid ounces) of chicken broth** and **4-6 ounces of uncooked noodles**. Then cover the soup pot, reduce the heat to medium-low and set the timer for 20 minutes.
5. Open the pot and add **2-3 cups diced or pulled apart, cooked chicken meat**, light and dark—skin discarded.
6. Add a pinch of **salt, pepper** and/or **garlic powder** to your taste. Cook 10 minutes longer.

Note: This is a great recipe to use up left-over chicken or grocery store Rotisserie chicken

Check out our handy grocery list on the next page to save you some time. Snap a picture of it with your Smart Phone and bring it with you on your shopping trip!

<u>Meal 4 Grocery List:</u>

- ☐ Whole grain wheat or white wheat bread
- ☐ Peanut butter (or sunflower butter, if a family member has a peanut allergy)
- ☐ Raisins or Banana
- ☐ Cucumbers
- ☐ Hummus (buy prepared at grocery store deli or make your own)
- ☐ 1% Milk

For Chicken Noodle Soup Recipe

- ☐ Olive or canola oil
- ☐ Celery
- ☐ Carrots
- ☐ Onion
- ☐ Fresh parsley
- ☐ Chicken broth
- ☐ Dry Noodles
- ☐ Cooked chicken meat, light and dark (without the skin)
- ☐ Pinch of salt, black pepper and garlic powder

NOTES:

____

____

____

____

____

____

____

Meal 5: Mediterranean Style Pizza

Mediterranean Style Pizza
Broccoli
Grapes
1% Milk or Water

Mediterranean Style Pizza Recipe (1 pizza):

1. Get out pizza crust and sheet pan.
2. Using the instructions on the **crust**, bake in the oven with Mediterranean-style toppings like red **pizza sauce** or **pesto sauce** + cut up **tomatoes** + chopped **sweet Bell peppers** + **olives** + fresh (or dried) **basil** + crumbled **feta cheese** (or Mozzarella.)
3. Cook according to instructions on the crust package.

Check out our handy grocery list on the next page to save you some time. Snap a picture of it with your Smart Phone and bring it with you on your shopping trip!

<u>Meal 5 Grocery List:</u>

- ☐ Fresh or frozen broccoli
- ☐ Grapes
- ☐ 1% Milk

For Pizza Recipe

- ☐ Pizza crust, thin style (buy crust at grocery store or make your own)
- ☐ Pizza sauce or Pesto sauce
- ☐ Tomatoes
- ☐ Sweet Bell peppers, any color
- ☐ Pitted olives
- ☐ Fresh or dried basil
- ☐ Feta cheese (or Mozzarella which is a milder flavor)

NOTES:

____

____

____

____

____

____

____

____

____

Meal 6: Turkey Burger on Bun

Turkey Burger on Bun
Sliced Tomato, Lettuce, Onion, Mustard, Light Mayo, Pickles
Baked Sweet Potato Fries
Orange or Tangerine
1% Milk or Water

Baked Sweet Potato Fries Recipe (4 servings):

1. Preheat oven to 425 degrees.
2. Scrub **2 medium sweet potatoes** (about 4 x 2 inches) with a vegetable brush under cool water. Do not peel the potatoes.
3. Using a cutting board and knife, cut potatoes into 3 x ½ inch 'sticks.'
4. Place into a bowl and add **1-2 teaspoons olive** or **canola oil**, then shake on **salt** and **pepper**.
5. Stir potato sticks to coat evenly with oil and seasonings.
6. Scatter them onto a flat sheet pan in a single layer.
7. Bake for 20-25 minutes.

Check out our handy grocery list on the next page to save you some time. Snap a picture of it with your Smart Phone and bring it with you on your shopping trip!

Meal 6 Grocery List:

- ☐ Turkey Burgers (buy frozen at grocery store or make your own)
- ☐ Burger Buns, whole wheat or white wheat, 3 inch size
- ☐ Sliced tomato, lettuce, onion
- ☐ Mustard, light mayo, pickles
- ☐ Oranges or Tangerines
- ☐ 1% Milk

For Baked Sweet Potato Fries Recipe

- ☐ Sweet potatoes, medium size
- ☐ Olive or canola oil
- ☐ Salt
- ☐ Black pepper

NOTES:

____

____

____

____

____

____

____

____

____

____

Meal 7: Whole Wheat Blueberry Pancakes with Turkey Sausage

Whole Wheat Blueberry Pancakes, with a little syrup
Turkey Sausage
Cut up Fruit (apples, cantaloupe and/or pears)
1% Milk or Water

Whole Wheat Blueberry Pancakes Recipe (8-10 pancakes):

1. Stir together **1 cup healthy pancake mix** with **1 cup whole wheat flour**.
2. Stir in **1 ¼ cups milk** and **1 egg**.
3. When smooth, add **1 cup fresh or frozen blueberries**. Stir gently to distribute berries evenly.
4. Using a ¼ cup measure for each pancake, ladle batter onto a medium-heated pan/griddle that is lightly sprayed with **cooking oil spray**.
5. Turn pancakes over when bubbles form, about 3 minutes per side.
6. Hold pancakes in the oven or toaster oven on warm heat.

Note: Pancakes reheat beautifully in the microwave oven on half power.

Check out our handy grocery list on the next page to save you some time. Snap a picture of it with your Smart Phone and bring it with you on your shopping trip!

- ☐ Syrup
- ☐ Turkey sausage
- ☐ Cut up fruit (apples, cantaloupe and/or pears)
- ☐ 1% Milk

For Whole Wheat Blueberry Pancakes Recipe

- ☐ Healthy Pancake & Baking Mix
- ☐ Whole wheat flour
- ☐ Milk, 1% or fat free skim
- ☐ Fresh or frozen blueberries
- ☐ Cooking oil spray
- ☐ Large egg

NOTES:

____

____

____

____

____

____

____

____

____

Meal 8: Grilled-in-the-Oven Fish

Grilled-in-Oven Fish with Bread Crumb Topping
Green Beans
Corn (frozen, canned or on-the-cob)
Yogurt & Mandarin Orange Parfait
1% Milk or Water

Grilled-In-Oven Fish Recipe (4 servings):

1. Preheat the oven to 400 degrees.
2. Get out an oven-safe sheet pan. Spray it lightly with **cooking oil spray** or cover it with parchment paper for easier clean-up.
3. Lay out **4 fish fillets**, about 4 ounces each, onto the pan with some space in-between.
4. In a small side bowl, mix **1-2 cups seasoned breadcrumbs** and **1-2 tablespoons extra virgin olive oil**.
5. Pile up the breadcrumbs on top of each fish fillet, then level out/pat down with a spoon so it sticks.
6. Drizzle a bit more olive oil on top of each fillet.
7. Bake for 8-10 minutes, keeping watch that the crumbs do not burn and fish cooks through.
8. Serve with a wedge of fresh **lemon**.

Check out our handy grocery list on the next page to save you some time. Snap a picture of it with your Smart Phone and bring it with you on your shopping trip!

<u>Meal 8 Grocery List:</u>

- ☐ Green beans
- ☐ Corn (frozen, canned or on-the-cob)
- ☐ Yogurt
- ☐ Mandarin oranges
- ☐ 1% Milk

For Grilled Fish Recipe

- ☐ Cooking oil spray
- ☐ Parchment paper (optional, to make cleanup easier)
- ☐ Fish fillets, fresh or frozen, thawed (ex. Flounder, tilapia, salmon, trout)
- ☐ Seasoned breadcrumbs (or make your own with a grater and stale bread)
- ☐ Extra virgin olive oil
- ☐ Salt and pepper to season
- ☐ Fresh lemon(s)

NOTES:

____

____

____

____

____

____

____

____

Meal 9: Spaghetti with Homemade Marinara Sauce

Spaghetti with Homemade Marinara (Red) Sauce & Meatballs
Shredded Lettuce Salad with cut up carrots & sweet red Bell
peppers, simple dressing
Italian Bread
Kiwi Fruit
1% Milk or Water

Homemade Marinara (Red) Sauce Recipe (4 servings):

1. Heat a medium-size skillet or frying pan on the stove to medium heat.
2. Place **2 tablespoons extra virgin olive oil** and **2 cloves crushed and minced garlic** into the pan.
3. When garlic begins to sizzle, cook about 2-3 minutes, stirring. Garlic will turn golden.
4. Add **2 cups crushed tomatoes**, **2 tablespoons water**, a pinch of **crushed red pepper flakes** (optional), a generous pinch of **salt** and black **pepper**, and **8 fresh basil leaves** torn into thirds (or 1 teaspoon dried basil) to the pan.
5. Cover pan with a lid and simmer over low heat, stirring once every 15 minutes.
6. Simmer sauce for 45-60 minutes to develop flavors.
7. Taste and adjust seasonings.

Homemade Meatballs Recipe – Look in Meal #1 (page 14)

Check out our handy grocery list on the next page to save you some time. Snap a picture of it with your Smart Phone and bring it with you on your shopping trip!

<u>Meal 9 Grocery List:</u>

- ☐ Spaghetti (try whole grain)
- ☐ Meatball ingredients (or keep it simple with lean hamburger rolled into 1-inch balls and baked)
- ☐ Lettuce (or buy it already shredded to save time)
- ☐ Carrots
- ☐ Sweet red Bell peppers
- ☐ Salad dressing
- ☐ Italian bread
- ☐ Kiwi fruit
- ☐ 1% Milk

For Homemade Marinara (Red) Sauce Recipe

- ☐ Extra virgin olive oil
- ☐ Garlic
- ☐ Canned crushed tomatoes
- ☐ Red pepper flakes (optional)
- ☐ Salt and black pepper
- ☐ Fresh basil leaves

NOTES:

____

____

____

____

____

____

____

____

Meal 10: Crispy Pan-Fried Chicken

Crispy Pan-Fried Chicken
(or substitute a grocery store rotisserie chicken)
Boiled Red Skin Potatoes
Sugar Snap Peas with Greek Yogurt Dip
Watermelon or In-Season Fruit
1% Milk or Water

Crispy Pan-Fried Chicken Recipe (4 servings)**:**

1. Mix up **1/4 cup flour**, 1/2 teaspoon **dried oregano**, ½ teaspoon **dried basil**, 1/8 teaspoon **crushed red pepper flakes** and 1/4 teaspoon **salt** in a shallow dish or on a dinner size plate.
2. Place **one egg** in a medium size bowl and whisk.
3. Mix **1 cup panko bread crumbs** and ¼ **cup grated Parmesan cheese** in a shallow dish or on a dinner size plate.
4. One at a time, dip **4 skinless and boneless chicken breast halves** into the flour mixture, then the egg, then the panko crumbs. Repeat this process with all the chicken.
5. Heat a large skillet or frying pan to medium heat.
6. Add **1 tablespoon canola or olive oil**, swirl it to cover bottom of pan, and place breaded chicken into pan.
7. Cook for about 2 minutes and add **1 more tablespoon oil**.
8. Turn chicken over, cover pan with a lid, and cook 4-5 minutes.
9. Turn chicken over again, cover pan with lid and cook 4-5 minutes.
10. Chicken is done when a meat thermometer test reads 170 degrees Fahrenheit.

<u>Meal 10 Grocery List:</u>

- ☐ Red skin potatoes
- ☐ Greek yogurt dip (or make your own)
- ☐ Sugar snap peas
- ☐ Watermelon or in-season fruit
- ☐ 1% Milk

For Crispy Pan-Fried Chicken Recipe

- ☐ Flour
- ☐ Dried oregano
- ☐ Dried basil
- ☐ Crushed red pepper flakes
- ☐ Salt
- ☐ Large egg
- ☐ Panko (Japanese) bread crumbs
- ☐ Grated Parmesan cheese
- ☐ Skinless, boneless chicken breast halves, 4-ounces
- ☐ Canola or Extra virgin olive oil

NOTES:

____

____

____

____

____

____

____

Meal 11: Stir-Fried Pork & Pineapple with Brown Rice

Stir Fried Pork & Pineapple
Brown Rice
Green Tossed Salad & Dressing
1% Milk or Water

Stir-Fried Pork & Pineapple Recipe (6 servings):

1. Heat a large wok or skillet to medium high heat and add **1/2 tablespoon canola oil.**
2. Add **1 pound pork tenderloin** cut into thin strips (about 3 inches x ¾ inch) and stir as it cooks, looking for a golden brown color.
3. After 3-4 minutes, push pork to one side of the wok/skillet or remove it to a plate.
4. Add **1/2 tablespoon canola oil, 1 cup broccoli florets, 1 cup snow peas, 1 cup carrots** and **1-2 cloves minced garlic** to the wok/skillet and stir.
5. Cook and stir vegetables about 3-4 minutes.
6. Add cooked pork back into vegetables in the wok/skillet and season with a mixture of **1-2 tablespoons soy sauce** and **1-2 tablespoons Hoisin sauce**.
7. Continue to cook and stir until vegetables are tender, about 2 more minutes.
8. At the last minute, add **1 cup drained pineapple chunks**. Sprinkle **2 chopped green onions** on top as a garnish.

Check out our handy grocery list on the next page to save you some time. Snap a picture of it with your Smart Phone and bring it with you on your shopping trip!

<u>Meal 11 Grocery List:</u>

- ☐ Brown Rice, instant (takes only 10 minutes to cook)
- ☐ Lettuce for green salad
- ☐ Salad dressing
- ☐ 1% Milk

For Stir-Fried Pork & Pineapple Recipe
- ☐ Canola oil
- ☐ Pork tenderloin, 1 pound makes 6 servings
- ☐ Broccoli florets, small
- ☐ Snow peas
- ☐ Baby carrots to slice into 'coins'
- ☐ Garlic, fresh or minced in a jar
- ☐ Soy sauce
- ☐ Hoisin sauce
- ☐ Fresh or canned pineapple, chunks/tidbits
- ☐ Green onions

NOTES:

____

____

____

____

____

____

____

____

Meal 12: English Muffin Pizza

English Muffin Pizza
Fresh Cut-Up Apple & Vanilla Yogurt Salad – mix together & chill
Celery Sticks with Peanut Butter
(or sunflower seed butter for peanut allergic kids)
1% Milk or Water

English Muffin Pizza Recipe (2 servings):

1. Separate **2 English Muffins** in half and lay out 4 halves flat on a sheet pan.
2. Spread **1 tablespoon tomato sauce** or pizza sauce onto each and then add **¼ cup chopped onions/mushrooms/sweet Bell peppers/diced lean ham** onto each.
3. Sprinkle a pinch of **dried basil** and **dried oregano** over top and finally sprinkle shredded **Mozzarella cheese** on the very top.
4. Bake at 350 degrees until cheese melts, about 6-8 minutes.

Check out our handy grocery list on the next page to save you some time. Snap a picture of it with your Smart Phone and bring it with you on your shopping trip!

<u>Meal 12 Grocery List:</u>

- ☐ Apples
- ☐ Vanilla yogurt
- ☐ Celery
- ☐ Peanut butter (or sunflower seed butter for peanut allergic kids)
- ☐ 1% Milk

For English Muffin Pizza Recipe

- ☐ English muffins, whole grain
- ☐ Canned tomato sauce or canned pizza sauce
- ☐ Vegetable toppings – onions, mushrooms, sweet Bell peppers
- ☐ Lean deli ham
- ☐ Dried basil
- ☐ Dried oregano
- ☐ Mozzarella cheese, shredded

NOTES:

____

____

____

____

____

____

____

____

____

Meal 13: Chicken & Cheese Quesadilla

Chicken & Cheese on Whole Wheat Quesadilla
(or try cooked shrimp & cheese)
Baked Corn Tortilla Chips
(use salsa and guacamole as tasty dips)
Fresh Mango
1% Milk or Water

Chicken & Cheese Quesadilla Recipe (2 servings):

1. Get out two **8-inch, whole wheat flour tortillas** and make a 'sandwich' with **½ cup chopped up cooked chicken** (or shrimp) and **¼ cup shredded cheddar cheese** in the middle.
2. Heat a large pan/skillet to medium heat and spray lightly with cooking oil spray.
3. Carefully lift the quesadilla (sandwich) into the heated skillet and cook for 4-5 minutes until golden brown.
4. Turn over and cook the other side until golden brown, about 4-5 minutes.
5. Remove quesadilla from pan and cut into 4- 6 triangles to serve. Each serving is ½ the 8-inch quesadilla 'sandwich.'
6. Serve with **salsa, avocado guacamole** and/or **hot sauce.** Ole!

Check out our handy grocery list on the next page to save you some time. Snap a picture of it with your Smart Phone and bring it with you on your shopping trip!

<u>Meal 13 Grocery List:</u>

- ☐ Baked Corn Tortilla Chips
- ☐ Fresh Mango
- ☐ 1% Milk

For Chicken, Cheese & Whole Wheat Quesadilla Recipe

- ☐ Whole wheat flour tortillas, 8 inch
- ☐ Cooked chicken (or, for another variation, try cooked shrimp)
- ☐ Cheddar cheese, shredded (or Mexican blend shredded cheese)
- ☐ Cooking oil spray
- ☐ Prepared salsa
- ☐ Prepared avocado guacamole (or make your own by adding garlic powder, fresh lemon juice, and a little salt to a mashed up ripe avocado)
- ☐ Hot sauce (optional)

NOTES:

____

____

____

____

____

____

____

____

Meal 14: Roast Beef & Mozzarella Roll-Ups

Roast Beef & Mozzarella Cheese Roll-Ups
Mustard, Light Mayo or Horseradish Sauce to dip
Yeast Roll
Sliced Cucumbers & Tiny Tomatoes
Oatmeal Cookie
1% Milk or Water

Roast Beef & Mozzarella Cheese Roll-Ups Recipe (2 servings):

1.   Get out a clean plate or cutting board.
2.   Lay down a flat slice of about **1-2 ounces lean roast beef** and then cover it with a slice of about **1 ounce Mozzarella cheese** (or, try Provolone cheese).
3.   Place a **pickle** wedge into the middle of each roll-up if you want to get fancy.
4.   Roll up the 2 layers, cut into 1 inch segments and secure each with a **tooth pick**.
5.   Use your favorite **mustard**, **light mayonnaise** and/or **horseradish sauce** as a tasty dip for the roll-ups.
6.   Each serving is 3-4 roll-ups.

Check out our handy grocery list on the next page to save you some time. Snap a picture of it with your Smart Phone and bring it with you on your shopping trip!

- ☐ Yeast rolls
- ☐ Cucumbers
- ☐ Tiny tomatoes
- ☐ Oatmeal cookie
- ☐ 1% Milk or water

For Roast Beef & Mozzarella Cheese Roll-Ups Recipe

- ☐ Cooked roast beef, 2 ounces for 2 servings
- ☐ Mozzarella cheese, 2 ounces for 2 servings
- ☐ Mustard, light mayo &/or horseradish sauce
- ☐ Pickle Wedges
- ☐ Toothpicks

NOTES:

____

____

____

____

____

____

____

____

____

Meal 15: Black Bean, Corn & Vegetable Wrap

Black Bean, Corn & Vegetable Wrap
Hummus and Baby Carrots
Super Easy Banana Smoothie

Black Bean, Corn & Vegetable Wrap Recipe (6 servings):

1. Lay out an **8-inch, whole grain wrap** or **flour tortilla** on a clean plate or cutting board.
2. In a separate bowl, mix together **1 cup drained, canned black beans, 1 cup drained, canned corn** (or thawed frozen corn), **1 cup chopped lettuce, ¼ cup minced onion, 1 cup chopped tomatoes**, and **¼ cup chopped fresh herbs** such as cilantro or parsley.
3. To the mixture, add the juice of **½ lime** and a pinch of **salt** and **garlic powder**. If you like a spicy wrap, add ¼-1/2 teaspoon of **crushed red pepper flakes**.
4. Mix all the wrap filling ingredients well and then measure 1 cup into the center of each wrap.
5. Roll up. Serve.

Super Easy Banana Smoothie Recipe (2 servings): Blend together **1-1/2 cups of 1% milk** and **1 ripe banana**.

Note: For a Banana-Chocolate Smoothie, add 1-2 teaspoons of unsweetened cocoa powder before blending.

Check out our handy grocery list on the next page to save you some time. Snap a picture of it with your Smart Phone and bring it with you on your shopping trip!

- ☐ Hummus (buy prepared at grocery store deli or make your own)
- ☐ Baby Carrots

For Black Bean, Corn & Vegetable Wrap Recipe
- ☐ Whole grain wrap or flour tortillas, 8-inch
- ☐ Canned black beans (or cook your own from dry)
- ☐ Canned corn (or frozen and let it thaw)
- ☐ Lettuce
- ☐ Onion
- ☐ Tomatoes
- ☐ Fresh cilantro or other favorite herb
- ☐ Fresh lime
- ☐ Garlic powder
- ☐ Salt
- ☐ Crushed red pepper flakes, optional

For Banana Smoothie Recipe
- ☐ 1% Milk
- ☐ Ripe Banana
- ☐ Unsweetened Cocoa Powder, optional

NOTES:

____

____

____

____

____

____

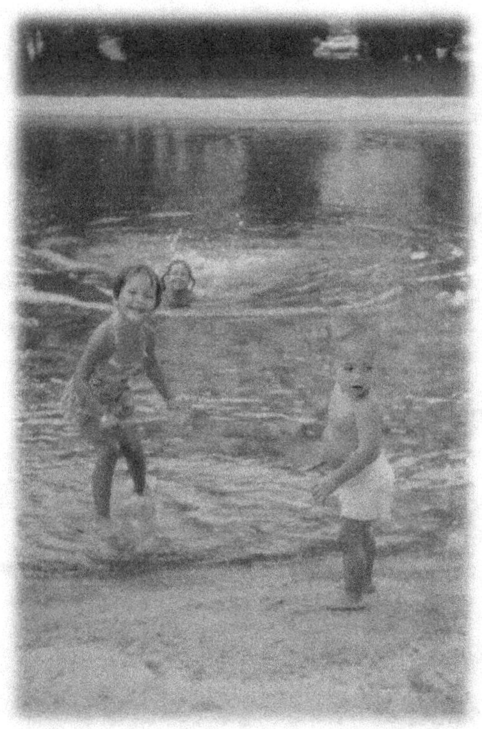

Eating More Vegetables

Vegetables don't always get along with kids – or adults. To encourage the friendship, relax and try these strategies. Even when it seems hopeless, keep trying because everyone needs to eat vegetables for good health, every meal and every day.

How Kids Benefit by Eating Vegetables
They…

- Feel better
- Stay healthier
- Grow up with more variety & balance on their plate
- Grow up willing to taste new foods
- Grow up to be teens, young adults and adults with fewer health problems

How Adults Benefit by Eating Vegetables

They...

- Feel better
- Stay healthier
- Enjoy more variety & balance on their plate
- Become adventurous with new foods
- Live their lives with fewer health problems

3 Places to Find Vegetables

When you consider the options, it's easy to find vegetables. Give kids permission to choose and keep an open mind as you look at all there is on display.

1. Explore the Grocery Store

Visit yourself or take your kids to the grocery store and study the salad bar choices. Take a self-serve container of something new to try at home.

- Fancy lettuce
- Shredded carrots
- Sliced mushrooms

2. Visit the Farmer's Market

Visit yourself or take your kids to a fresh-air Farmer's Market and study the choices. Bring along a reusable shopping bag as you choose what to buy. Take home a few vegetables.

- Purple carrots
- Sweet potatoes
- Rainbow Swiss chard
- Small white turnips

3. Be a Farmer

Go yourself or take your kids to a pick-your-own farm, or grow your own back yard vegetable garden. Enjoy your harvest. Take home vegetables to try.

- Sugar snap peas
- Green beans
- Tomatoes
- Pumpkin or an acorn squash

- ♥ **Bright idea!** *Vegetable outings always go smoother when kids and adults dress down with blue jeans, comfy closed-toe shoes and a hat for the sun.*

6 Ways to Prep and Eat Vegetables

When kids and adults begin to add more vegetables to their meals and snacks, it becomes a new-normal for what to expect. Try these strategies to encourage more vegetables on your table and into your mouth.

1. **Roast fresh vegetables - for a sweet flavor and tender texture. Try roasting these (check our Roasted Veggies recipe on page 102):**
    - Butternut squash chunks
    - Green beans
    - Asparagus
    - Sweet or white potato fries
    - Okra (Hint: Roast it whole, not cut up)
    - Zucchini
2. **Dip vegetables into a sauce or dip**
    - Hummus
    - Ranch dressing (Easy recipe: Mix nonfat Greek yogurt + dry packet of Ranch dressing spices from grocery store)

- Honey mustard (Easy recipe: Mix 2 tablespoons mustard with 1 tablespoon honey)
- Gochujang Korean sauce – (Hint: Find this spicy, traditional sauce in the International Foods Aisle of the grocery store, or an Asian specialty grocery store)

3. **Offer vegetables raw and cooked**
    - Grated carrots
    - Yellow squash spears
    - Sweet Bell pepper strips (red, orange, yellow, purple)
    - Cucumber rounds
    - Jicama (Most kids like it raw, cut into 'stick' shapes the best)
    - Snow peas
    - Sugar snap peas

4. **Make a guessing game of it**
    - Broccoli forest – steamed broccoli florets lined up on a plate with stems resting in a bed of hummus and dusted with paprika for colorful dipping
    - Carrot curls – curly Qs made with a carrot peeler and a long carrot. Kids can eat it with their fingers, raw or steamed and cooled. (Hint: As you cut the carrots, drop them into a bowl of icy cold water to preserve the orange color.)
    - Sweet potato 'dip sticks' – raw, peeled (or not) sweet potatoes made into 'stick' shapes and then stuck into a small dish of light cream cheese to dip
    - Ants on a log – 3 inch pieces of celery with peanut (or sunflower) butter filling the center hollow and decorated on top with raisins or dried cherries

5. **Blend it**
   - Creamy potato or tomato soup
   - Super smooth mashed white potatoes or sweet potatoes (with or without garlic or garlic powder added for a kick)
   - Butternut squash soup
   - Avocado guacamole (Easy recipe: Blend ripe avocado with a splash of fresh lemon or lime juice and a pinch of salt)
   - Green smoothie (Easy recipe: Blend 3-5 strawberries, fresh or frozen + ½ ripe banana + ½ cup orange juice + handful fresh spinach) Kids love it when you call this a Shrek Smoothie!

6. **Stir-fry it**
   - Cut up or grate an apple or pear and add to the vegetables in any stir-fry to add nature's sweetness
   - Drizzle a teaspoon of honey into any stir-fry to sweeten it up

Vegetable Recipes that Kids Like

- **Roasted Rainbow Vegetables** – Check out our recipe for colorful, sweet-tasting, cooked veggies on page 102.
- **Broccoli with Cheese**– Check out our recipe for cooked broccoli the healthy way on page 96.
- **Bunny Rabbit Salad**– Check out our recipe for a carrot side dish that tastes like dessert on page 99.

A Family Club to Encourage Kids to Eat Their Vegetables

Parents can inspire their kids to eat vegetables and kids can inspire their parents, too.

1. Once a week, have a veggie tasting at the dinner table.
2. Make a rule that everyone in the family – parent and kids – will taste everything.
3. Taste, raise hands to vote on who likes the featured veggie.
4. If there is a tie vote, then bring the same veggie to another tasting in a couple weeks and vote again.
5. If more than half the family votes 'yes', then add the veggie to next week's meal plan and grocery shopping list.
6. Be sure to keep a list or picture chart of veggies tried and veggies liked.

Bright idea! *If you're a parent, do your very best to always talk about vegetables in positive words with your kids. For example, use words like these: crunchy, tasty, colorful, sweet, awesome, delicious, healthy.*

Snack Time

A well-planned snack can make the difference between a cranky melt-down and a happy day. Let's be honest, even adults sometimes lose it and can benefit from a well-timed, nutritious snack. A smart snack choice is something that's full of nutrition, practical for you, and totally delicious. Here are 25 snacks to try at home, after school, on the sports field, at the office, or on a car trip.

25 Modern Snacks

Featuring Fresh Fruits & Vegetables

- Apple slices with sunflower butter to dip
- Small banana with 1% milk
- Celery sticks with light (Neufchatel) herb-flavored cream cheese to dip
- Orange or clementine with almonds
- Cut up pineapple & plain or vanilla yogurt
- Baby carrots with vanilla yogurt to dip
- Cucumber slices spread with light (Neufchatel) cream cheese
- Sweet Bell pepper strips with hummus to dip
- Grape tomatoes with cubes of cheese
- Cantaloupe cubes wrapped up with a small piece of lean ham

Featuring Grain Foods

- Corn tortilla spread with vegetarian refried black beans & sprinkled with cheese
- Whole grain crackers with applesauce to dip (unsweetened applesauce is best)
- Whole grain crackers spread with light (Neufchatel) cheese & topped with a mandarin orange slice
- Oat cereal with raisins & 1% milk
- Oatmeal granola with plain or vanilla yogurt
- Baked corn tortilla chips with avocado guacamole to dip
- Half tuna salad sandwich on whole wheat or white wheat bread
- Half egg salad sandwich on whole wheat or white wheat bread
- Peanut butter & sliced banana wrap on small, whole wheat tortilla
- Dried cranberries mixed with cashews and popcorn in a small container

Featuring Dairy Foods

- Cheese melted onto whole grain toast, English muffin half or a whole wheat tortilla
- String cheese & grapes
- 1% Cottage cheese with canned fruit (fruit canned in its own juice is best)
- Plain or vanilla yogurt layered with berries (fresh or partly thawed frozen berries are great)
- Blender smoothie made from ¾ cup 1% milk + ½ large, ripe banana + 1 teaspoon Cocoa powder

♥ **Bright Idea!** *Check out our <u>Safety Tips</u> to make sure your kids are old enough to eat these snacks safely.*

Easy & Fun Theme Dinners

In a world that's become crazy-busy, dinnertime can be prime time for spending quality moments with the entire family. Instead of dinner being a chore, set aside some time and make it an hour of bonding, teaching and having fun with a nutritious meal.

For each month, there is a theme dinner and four kid-activity options to choose from. Select one or do all of them. Make your main goals to gather your family, spark imaginations, get conversations flowing and embrace and enjoy a tasty meal.

Keep in mind that every plan can be tweaked for your family. For example, you can prepare your activities a few days beforehand or get everything together on theme dinner night. Also, remember to choose an activity that best fits your child's personality and your patience. These are short and easy ways to keep your kids busy while you prepare dinner.

Kid-Activity Options for Theme Dinners

- Crafters (for kids with busy hands)
- Artists (for kids who are more visual)
- Writers (for kids who prefer to use letters and words to communicate)
- Cooks (for kids who are ready to learn in the kitchen)

♥ **Bright Idea!** *An excellent way to get your kids even more excited and involved in your theme dinner is through their peers. Talk to the teacher about it and see if she/he will expand on the idea with the entire class.*

January: It's a New Year

Start off the New Year with a little humor. Can your kids guess the theme after they see the menu?

Menu:

- **NEW York Steak** Grill or broil to the doneness you like.
- **NEW Potatoes** Wash and cut potatoes in halves or fourths. Toss with olive oil and a favorite seasoning. Roast on a sheet pan in a single layer at 425 degrees for 20-25 minutes.
- **Santa Fe Black Beans with Salsa** (from NEW Mexico. Get it?) Drain canned black beans and add a spoonful of salsa.
- **NEW Year's Broccoli** Steam or microwave until tender. Sprinkle with shredded cheese.

Activity: NEWspaper Placemats highlighting the past year. Cut Poster Board for each placemat or use a blank piece of any color paper.

Crafters: Have kids cut out pictures from newspapers or magazines and paste them on their posterboard placemat (glue sticks equal less mess). At dinner, discuss the pictures and why they chose them.

Artists: Have kids draw pictures of family adventures from the past year onto their placemat. At dinner, relive your memories as the kids explain why they chose them.

Writers: On their placemat, have kids write a short article about your family adventures as if for a newspaper. At dinner, talk over a bonus article they can write about the upcoming year. Older kids can do this on their own during the week. It's a great keepsake when repeated each year.

Cooks: Depending on their skill level, pick an activity that is safe and fun for kids:

- Slice new potatoes in halves or fourths.
- Toss potatoes in olive oil.
- Sprinkle herbs onto the cut potatoes.
- Wash the broccoli.
- Cut up the broccoli.
- Sprinkle shredded cheese on the cooked broccoli.
- Stir up the black beans and salsa.

NOTES:

____

____

____

____

____

____

____

____

February: The Red Month & Healthy Hearts

It's all about hearts and the color red during February with Valentine's Day and the national celebration of Healthy Heart Month!

<u>**Menu:**</u>

- **RED Sauce over Spaghetti** (see recipe on page 30)
- **Tossed Salad with RED Radishes & Tomatoes**
- **RED Strawberry & Vanilla Yogurt Layered Parfait**
  Everyone can make their own!

<u>**Activities:**</u> Valentine's Day Cards and a Restaurant Menu that's Healthy for the Heart

Crafters: Have kids cut out heart shapes in any color paper. Help kids write a Valentine's Day message in the center. Tear tissue paper into small pieces and crumple into balls. Glue crumpled paper onto cards to decorate. Or, color with crayons.

Artists: Have kids fold any color paper in half. For the front of the menu, kids can draw a name and logo for their restaurant. On the inside, kids can draw pictures of the dinner menu items. Decorate with Valentine's Day stickers or crumpled tissue paper balls. Or, get out crayons for kids to draw.

Writers: Have kids create a restaurant menu with heart health facts. List the facts on the menu cover. Older kids can create a few extra menus with heart healthy foods to serve later in the month.

Cooks: Depending on their skill level, pick an activity that is safe and fun for kids.

- Heat and stir the sauce.
- Wash the lettuce for salad. Tear into bite size pieces.
- Prepare salad with radishes and tomatoes.
- Cap the strawberries.
- Slice the strawberries, tomatoes and radishes
- Layer the yogurt parfait.
- Serve plates with spaghetti and spoon on the sauce.
- Shake on the Parmesan.

Bonus RED Game: Spend a few minutes during dinner to see who can list the most foods that are red. Will the winner get out of cleaning up after dinner?

NOTES:

____

____

____

____

____

____

____

____

____

March: Go Green for St. Patrick's Day

Grab a little luck of the Irish by eating fun, green food and planning a spring garden!

Menu:

- **GREEN Eggs and Ham** (Add 1-2 drops of food-grade blue food coloring into your eggs then scramble them up to make green)
- **GREEN Cabbage Coleslaw**
- **GREEN Basil Pesto on Pasta**
- **GREEN Drink** (Add a drop of food-grade green food coloring to a glass of 1% milk)

Activities: Real Vegetable Stamps, Limericks and A Spring Garden

Crafters and Artists: Make placemats on white paper using real vegetable stamps. Slice a green pepper in half (top-to-bottom) and dip in green, washable paint to make Shamrock shapes. Slice an okra through the middle, side-to-side, to make flower stamps.

Writers: Write a funny limerick about each family member but don't add their name. During dinner, see who can guess the 'star' of each limerick. Here's one to spark your kids' imagination:

> *There once was an apple named Al*
> *Who complained to be nothing but chow.*
> *He learned how to sing;*
> *His voice had a nice zing.*
> *Alas he had no legs to bow.*

Cooks: Depending on their skill level, pick an activity that is safe and fun for kids.

- Add shredded cabbage, salt, pepper, and light mayo to a bowl to make coleslaw. Stir it up.
- Crack fresh eggs and scramble them in a bowl.
- Add food coloring to eggs and drinks.
- Stir scrambled eggs while they cook.
- Slice ham.
- Stir the basil pesto into cooked and drained pasta.

- ♥ **Bright Idea!** *Mix a few drops of green food coloring with water and freeze in ice cubes trays for lime colored ice to add to your beverage.*
- ♥ **Bright Idea!** *Talk over a spring garden including where yours will be (sunny back yard or flower pots) and what you will plant. Radish seeds, onion sets, and a small parsley plant are a great starting point.*

NOTES:

____

____

____

____

____

____

April: Spring Colors & Traditions

A colorful Chinese Stir-Fry and the Zodiac calendar are fun for kids!

<u>**Menu:**</u>

- **SPRING Roll** (buy the kind you can bake in the oven <u>or</u> drop by the Chinese take-out)
- **SPRING Onions Stir-Fry** (combine spring onions with colorful sweet Bell peppers, snow peas and chicken)
- **Rice**
- **SPRING Strawberries & Cream** (slice up the berries and then let kids spray on some real whipped cream)

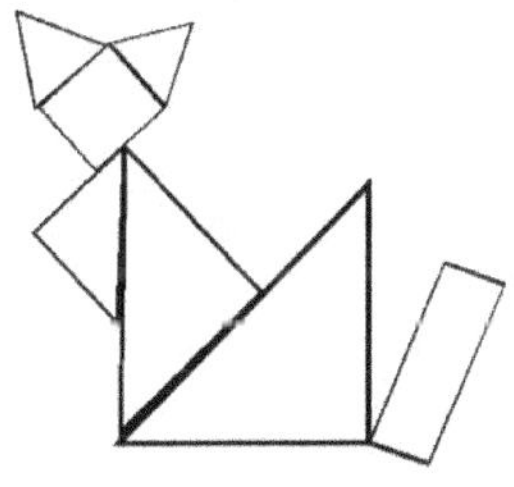

Cat Tangram

<u>**Activities:**</u> Chinese Traditional Crafts and the Zodiac

Crafters: Create Tangram animals. Cut out various shapes (older kids can do this part) and have kids use patterns to create creatures. Numerous templates can be found online.

Artists: Make Chinese Placemats with Zodiac animals. Older kids can research the signs for each family member's personalized placemat.

Writers: Have kids write Chinese cookie-style fortunes on small slips of paper, place in a bowl and then take turns drawing fortunes during dinner. To spark ideas, use kids' books or a book of quotes.

Cooks: Depending on their skill level, pick an activity that is safe and fun for kids.

- Wash vegetables for stir fry.
- Slice vegetables for stir fry.
- Cook stir fry.
- Serve cooked rice.
- Prepare dipping sauces for spring rolls.
- Spoon strawberries into individual dessert bowls.

- ♥ **Bright Idea!** *Turn it into a movie night and Watch Kung Fu Panda, The Amazing Panda Adventure or The Karate Kid remake after dinner.*

NOTES:

____

____

____

____

____

____

____

May: Memorial Day Celebration

Help your kids appreciate and love America as summer gets started.

Menu:

- **Spinach FLAG Pizza**—see recipe below
- **FREEDOM Fries** – Otherwise known as Baked Sweet Potato Fries (see our recipe on page 24)
- **PATRIOTIC Parfait** – Layers of vanilla yogurt with blueberries and strawberries

Spinach Flag Pizza: Lightly spray a rectangular sheet pan with vegetable oil spray. Roll out premade grocery store rectangular pizza dough (look in the dairy section) onto the sheet pan. Spread on a thin layer of pizza sauce then sprinkle with dried basil and oregano. Lay out a light layer of spinach in the upper left hand corner in a square shape. Dot the spinach section with Mozzarella cheese for stars. Then, add flag stripes on the rest of the pizza alternating between sliced plum tomatoes and Mozzarella cheese. Bake according to instructions on the pizza crust package.

- ♥ **Bright Idea!** *If you can't find rectangular pizza dough, outline a rectangular flag shape with cheese on top of a circular premade crust.*

Activities: Streamers, Thank You Cards and Colorful Placemats

Crafters: Have kids make star streamers from red and blue construction paper (younger kids may need a little hand with this task). Or, kids may want white stars to color themselves. Make small holes on the tip of each star, then thread each star onto yarn or dental floss, tying a knot after each star to keep it steady. Hang the streamers across the meal table.

Artists and Writers: Have kids make cards for veterans. Write the words, "Thank you for…" on the outside and, on the inside, write FREEDOM down the left side. Have kids draw pictures of what freedom means to them or a word for each letter. For example, 'Family' for the 'F' in Freedom. Or, challenge older kids to make meaningful words from each letter.

Cooks: Depending on their skill level, pick an activity that is safe and fun for kids.

- Roll out pizza dough to lay in the sheet pan.
- Prepare pizza toppings by washing, slicing and shredding.
- Scrub the sweet potatoes with a vegetable brush & cool water in the kitchen sink.
- Wash blueberries and strawberries.
- Cap and slice strawberries.
- Layer the dessert parfaits.

- ♥ **Bright Idea!** *If it's a nice, warm day in May then set up your theme dinner in the back yard, on the deck, or at the neighborhood park.*

NOTES:

____

____

____

____

____

____

June: Summer Picnics Make Kids Smile

Summertime is a celebration of family, friends, yard games and tasty finger foods for a picnic! To get the kids moving, go with a rowdy game of tag, one-on-one soccer or some Frisbee fun.

Menu:

- **Finger Sandwiches** (peanut butter and honey, cucumber and hummus, or turkey and cheese)
- **Deviled Eggs** (use light mayonnaise <u>or</u> a mix of mayo and plain Greek yogurt)
- **Carrots, Celery, Sweet Bell Pepper Strips**
- **Melon Kabobs**
- **Less Sugary Lemonade** (see recipe on page 2)

Activities: DIY Picnic Games and Nature Art

Crafters: Have kids cut a hole in a paper plate and then hang the loop from a tree branch. Kids can take turns trying to toss a ball through the hole....and adults, too.

Artists: Have kids pack up and bring their art supplies and a clipboard to hold their paper. Then, pick an outdoor scene for them to draw from the picnic site.

Writers: Have kids take turns describing something at the picnic with 3-4 words and see who can guess it. For example, these words—ringed, swaying, gnarled, slender—could be used to describe a tree. Have older kids take it a step further and write a short poem about something at the picnic using as many descriptive words as they can.

Cooks: Depending on their skill level, pick an activity that is safe and fun for kids.

- Cut bread for sandwiches into small squares.
- Make finger sandwiches.
- Peel eggs after cooling them.
- Prepare deviled egg mixture.
- Stuff deviled eggs.
- Arrange cut up vegetables on a platter.
- Cut melon into cubes or balls.
- Assemble melon kabobs.
- Stir lemonade.

♥ **Bright Idea!** *Be super smart about food safety in the summer heat. Load cold foods into an insulated cooler with plenty of ice to transport it to your picnic site. Leave foods sitting out of the cooler for no longer than 1 hour before packing them back into the cooler. Replace the ice if it melts.*

NOTES:

____

____

____

____

____

____

____

July: Bring on the Beach

Celebrate summer with a beach themed meal, either at the beach or at home. For extra fun, have the kids wear their swim suits to the dinner table.

Menu:

- **FISH Sandwich**
- **WATERmelon**
- **SUNflower Seeds**
- **Kiwi-Blueberry SEAWATER** Create an aqua color by adding slices of kiwi and/or blueberries into glasses of ice water

Activities: Beachy Table Centerpiece, Decorated Beach Balls and Poems

Crafters: Have kids craft a beachy centerpiece on a baking sheet of sand. If sand is not practical, play dough is another option that can easily be made at home. A quick internet search brings up many easy methods.   Try mixing 2 cups warm water, 2 cups flour, 1 cup of salt and 2 tablespoons of cooking oil. Add food coloring or glitter for fun color and sparkles.

- ♥ **Bright Idea!** *Magnetic sand - found at craft stores - is a great alternative to real beach sand for crafting.*

Artists: Have kids decorate beach balls (from your $1 store) using permanent markers. Encourage them to draw beachy pictures like the sun, fish, sea birds, waves or sand castles.

- ♥ **Bright Idea!** *Permanent markers are permanent. So it's best to do this activity outdoors in play clothes. If the marking gets out of hand, rubbing alcohol can dilute the ink.*

Writers: Have kids write beachy poems to read during dinner. Encourage them to use words that rhyme with beach, sand, fish, bird and sun. Adults can join in, too, for some silly fun.

Cooks: Depending on their skill level, pick an activity that is safe and fun for kids.

- Cook the fish.
- Create the fish sandwich with toppings and assemble it.
- Make watermelon balls with a scoop.
- Put sunflower seeds into little cups.
- Place slices of kiwi and/or blueberries into the water glasses.

♥ **Bright Idea!** *After dinner, take advantage of the longer evenings and bop a beach ball back-and-forth. Can you keep it from touching the ground?!*

NOTES:

____

____

____

____

____

____

____

August: A Fun Alphabet Dinner

A transition from summer to school is smoother with 'sneak peeks' of fun learning throughout August. An alphabet dinner goes with any letters, and we're starting with A, B, C.

<u>Menu:</u>

- **Bison Burger on Bun** (Local high end grocery stores may have this. If not, opt for lean ground beef.)
- **Asparagus** (See our recipe on page 102 for roasting tips)
- **Bunny Rabbit Salad** (see our recipe on page 99)
- **Cantaloupe**
- **Chocolate Milk** (Mix 1% chocolate milk half-and-half with 1% white milk for less sugar.)

<u>Activities:</u> Baking the A, B, Cs, Alphabet Placemats and Tongue Twisters

<u>Crafters:</u> Have kids play with their food. Buy breadstick dough, then have kids shape it into the letters A, B and C. Add these to your menu or save for tomorrow's breakfast.

<u>Artists:</u> Have kids make paper placemats by drawing and coloring foods that begin with the letters A, B and C.

<u>Writers:</u> Have kids create food themed tongue twisters or tiny alliterative sentences with A, B, and C. See how many times you can speak these without laughing:

- Apes ate apples.
- Bears bonk bananas.
- Crickets crave crepes.

<u>Cooks:</u> Depending on their skill level, pick an activity that is safe and fun for kids.

- Mix seasonings into ground bison and shape into burgers.
- Rinse asparagus in cool water.

- Break tough stem ends off of asparagus, or cut off ends carefully.
- Cook asparagus.
- Rinse off cantaloupe in cool water.
- Slice or use melon scoop on the cantaloupe.
- Stir up the chocolate milk.

NOTES:

____

____

____

____

____

____

____

____

September: Johnny Appleseed & Fall Apples

Celebrate John Chapman, AKA Johnny Appleseed, who was born September 26, 1774. He was a conservationist and a great guy who spread the growth of apple trees across the Midwest.

Menu:

- **Pancakes with APPLEsauce** (make pancakes, then top with applesauce for a healthy twist)
- **APPLE Sausage**
- **Hard Boiled Eggs**
- **Fresh Apple Salad** (see our recipe on page 103)

Activities: Decorated Lunch Bags, Fancy Pancake Shapes and An-Apple-a-Day Banners

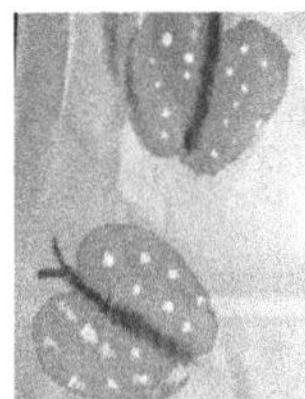

Crafters: Have kids make butterfly lunch bags with apple stamps. Slice apple in half, paint cut side, and gently press onto paper. Let dry for a few minutes and add body, head and colorful spots.

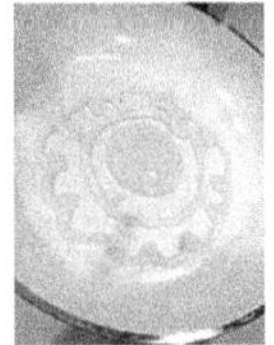

Artists: Have kids put the pancake mix in a squirt bottle and make different designs in the pancake pan. Let the design cook for 30-45 seconds, then fill in. Flip when ready. Be sure to closely supervise this activity.

- ♥ **Bright Idea:** *Make plain pancakes first and hold them in the oven or toaster oven on warm heat. Then, make one 'designer pancake' as above for every member of the family.*

Writers: Make An-Apple-a-Day banners for the kitchen or dining room. List the benefits of eating apples on construction paper or paper you have recycled. During dinner, flip over the banners and see who can name the most apple ideas -- without peeking.

Cooks: Depending on their skill level, pick an activity that is safe and fun for kids.

- Stir pancake mix.
- Cook pancakes.
- Top pancakes with applesauce.
- Peel the cooled, hard boiled eggs.
- Get out the ingredients and stir the apple salad.

NOTES:

____

____

____

____

____

____

____

____

____

October: Halloween Month is Here

Have a little fun with a spooky holiday and not-so-scary menu. Get everyone in the family to wear a funny hat to the dinner table, or a mask over their eyes - not mouths.

Menu:

- **MUMMY Dogs** (Wrap pre-cooked turkey sausage mummy-style with whole grain crescent dough and bake according to package instructions. Use mustard or ketchup dots for eyes.)
- **BLACK CAT Carrot & Cucumber Slices with HALLOWEEN Black Bean Hummus Dip**
- **Banana GHOSTS on a Stick** (Skewer bananas on a popsicle stick. Use mini chocolate chips for eyes and mouth.)
- **PUMPKIN Seeds**

- ♥ **Bright Idea!** *Keep your Jack-o-Lantern's seeds. Then either dry and save them for planting next spring or roast them for a tasty & nutritious snack now. Wash, dry and scatter pumpkin seeds on a sheet pan. Spray them lightly with vegetable oil spray, then sprinkle with a favorite seasoning such as salt, chili powder, garlic powder or cinnamon. Roast in the oven or toaster oven at 375 degrees for about seven minutes. Keep a close eye on them and remove when they're golden brown.*

Activities: Spooky Eyes, Halloween Haiku, Pumpkin Faces and Cat Faces

Crafters: Have kids make spooky eyes to hide in the bushes or around the house using toilet paper rolls. Cut eye holes in the center and insert a glow stick (from your $1 store). Twist edges shut. Spooky!

For the Cat Faces, use sliced cucumber circles for the face and curled carrot strips for the whiskers. Black bean hummus dip can be dotted on with a toothpick for the eyes and spooky smile.

Artists: Have kids draw pumpkin faces on oranges using permanent markers. Put the decorated oranges into a bowl for a creative centerpiece.

Writers: Have kids write a Halloween Haiku which is a Japanese poem made up of three lines, generally broken into 5, 7, and 5 syllables. These unique poems are a simple and fun way to express nature using sensory language. Can you guess what this Haiku is about?

Silent, smooth, orange gourd.
Slice it, scoop it and carve it,
Smiling light greets guests!

Cooks: Depending on their skill level, pick an activity that is safe and fun for kids.

- Wrap mummy dogs with whole grain crescent dough.
- Dot eyes on mummy dogs after they are cooked.
- Assemble the banana ghosts.
- Sort, wash and dry the pumpkin seeds.
- Sprinkle seasoning(s) on pumpkin seeds (experiment with different flavors on one pan).

- ♥ **Bright Idea!** *Use cooked fresh pumpkin pulp in Italian marinara sauce, muffins, or soups throughout the year or save time by using cooked canned 100% pure pumpkin. All pumpkin is very nutritious.*

November: Pilgrims' Dinner with a Modern Twist

Turkey, potatoes, corn, and pumpkin pie are foods we eat today for a special Thanksgiving dinner. But, what was on the table at the very first Thanksgiving? History tells us that the original menu included turkey, waterfowl such as duck and goose, venison, fish, lobster, clams, berries, fruit, pumpkin and squash.

Try our menu for a fun way to merge Thanksgiving history with today's more modern traditions.

<u>Menu:</u>

- **Baked Turkey Legs or Grilled Tilapia**
- **Roasted Root Vegetables** (see our recipe on page 102)
- **Sliced Fall Pears & Apples**
- **Easy Pumpkin Pie** (see our recipe on page 104)

<u>Activities</u>: Nature's Table Decoration, Hand Turkey Placemats and Thankful Thoughts

Crafters: Have kids collect outdoor treasures like pinecones, colorful leaves, stones, or whatever catches their eye. Let them artfully arrange the objects in the center of the table.

- ♥ **Bright Idea!** *For easy clean up, place newspaper or an extra tablecloth underneath their centerpiece.*

Artists: Help kids make handprint turkey placemats. Trace kids' hands to make a turkey body with the thumb as its neck and fingers as its feathers. Add small legs. Have the kids trace their hands in various poses to create different turkeys, then color and decorate with Pilgrim hats and other fall décor.

Writers: Have kids pass out slips of paper to all dinner guests who can then write down a few things for which they're thankful. Fold the papers, place them into a bowl and then choose someone to select the notes and read aloud. Who can guess the guest who wrote each thankful note?

Cooks: Depending on their skill level, pick an activity that is safe and fun for kids.

- Season the fish or turkey.
- Wash the vegetables.
- Peel the carrots.
- Cut vegetables into 1-inch chunks.
- Season the vegetables with a little olive oil, salt and pepper.
- Put seasoned vegetables onto a sheet pan.
- Add pumpkin pie ingredients into the blender.

- ♥ **Bright Idea!** *Since togetherness and interaction are important, stay at the table after dinner and play a game like 'spoons' with cards or another family favorite.*

NOTES:

____

____

____

____

____

____

____

December: Let it Snow

Kids get excited when they hear the word...snow! This dinner will remind everyone of snow whether they live in northern Canada, North Carolina or Miami Beach.

<u>Menu:</u>

- **Ground Turkey Meatballs** Sprinkled with Parmesan (see our recipe on page 14)
- **SNOW-Y Mashed Potatoes**
- **Roasted Cauliflower SNOWballs** (see our recipe on page 102)
- **Grape SNOWmen Skewers** (Skewer 2 light green seedless grapes for the body and 1 red seedless grape as the head onto a long toothpick; See Safety Tips on page 8.)

<u>Activities</u>: Grape Snowmen, Shaving Cream Paintings and Indoor Activity Bucket

Crafters: Have kids put together the grape snowmen using long toothpicks or short skewers. Decorate using broken pretzels for arms and mini chocolate chips pushed in, point first, for eyes and/or buttons.

Artists: Have kids make shaving cream paintings. Mix equal parts white foam shaving cream and glue and then add glitter and/or food coloring for sparkly shades. Have kids experiment by spreading the 'goo' with paint brushes, spoons or sponges for cool effects. Snow art dries into puffy 3-D pictures.

Writers: Have kids make an indoor activity bucket. On small pieces of paper, have kids write down inside activity ideas. Add some items needed into the bucket such as:

- Stopwatch (great way to see how many jumping jacks can be done in one minute, how many times they can run back and forth down the hall or how long they can juggle 2-3 oranges)
- Dice (take turns rolling how many times to do a certain activity like hopping, twisting or singing a song)
- Deck of cards
- Small ball

♥ **Bright Idea!** *Save the bucket. Whenever the kids complain that there's nothing to do, have them pick out an idea.*

Cooks: Depending on their skill level, pick an activity that is safe and fun for kids.

- Mix ground turkey breast with seasoning and bread crumbs (or uncooked oats).
- Shape the meatballs.
- Peel the potatoes.
- Mash the potatoes.
- Rinse cauliflower in cool water and break apart the flowers.
- Put the cauliflower flowers on a sheet pan.
- Wash the grapes.
- Assemble the grape snowmen.

♥ **Bright Idea!** *After dinner, draw an indoor activity idea from the bucket and play together!*

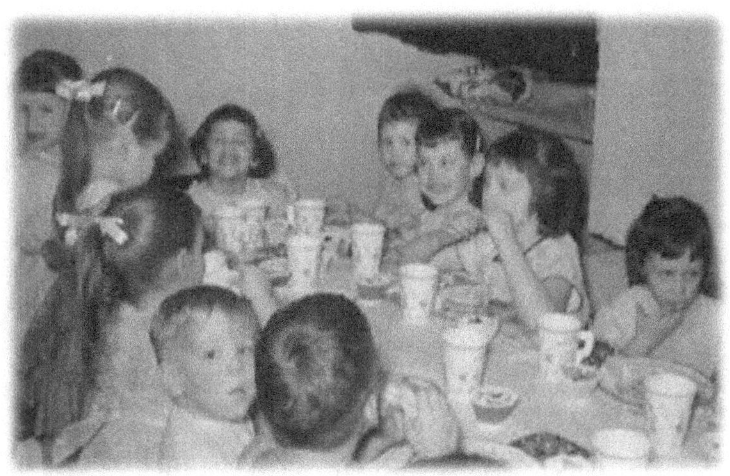

Modern Party Planning

We all like a party. Yet, coming up with ideas can be really challenging. These party planners are designed to save you time, money, and to make it possible to entertain easily at home. There are three fun themes, each with its own menu, decorations, activities and invitation.

If you're feeling really motivated, you could use one of our party ideas as a theme dinner and prepare throughout the week— with the kids' help, of course.

- Robin Hood Party
- Jungle Animal Party
- Classic Games Party

Robin Hood Party

This is a magical tale of adventure that takes place in Sherwood Forest and Nottingham Castle. It's an easy theme to tailor to boys, girls, or both.

Menu

- **The Forest:** Create a hummus river lined with standing broccoli florets. Dip and dipper – voila!
- **Archery Targets:** Place a grape tomato in the middle of pineapple rings to make fruit bullseyes.
- **Turkey Legs:** Bake or grill the leg part of chicken wings as kid-sized 'turkey legs.' Before cooking, brush legs with barbecue sauce to add a flavor most kids enjoy.
- **Target Cupcakes:** Make our Chocolate-y Banana Cupcakes (see recipe on page 98) ahead of time and have party kids decorate their own cupcakes like targets with tubed icing.

Decorations

- **Forest:** Hang brown and green streamers around the party room and use earthy colors for your tablecloth, napkins and plates to create Sherwood Forest ambiance.
- **Fort:** Use huge appliance boxes to create a fort or drape bed sheets over strings tied between chairs in the party room.
- **Trees:** Cut out trunk shapes from cardboard and tape them to the walls. During the party, have blindfolded guests play 'Pin the Leaves on the Tree' with tape attached to cut leaf shapes.
- **Castle:** Cut a door and windows into an appliance box for Nottingham Castle. As party kids arrive, get them

started with decorating the castle with crayons, stickers and tissue paper as window curtains.

- ♥ **Bright Idea!** *Many appliance stores have refrigerator and stove boxes to donate so be sure to ask for them. Call early in the morning to see what is available.*

Activities

Keep the kids busy with these:

- **Robin Hood T-shirts:** Cut neck and waist in V-pattern and let kids decorate their shirts with t-shirt markers from a local craft store. Tie around their waist with twine.
- **Treasure Hunt:** Depending on how much space you have, keep this game small or larger.
    1. Hide pennies in a sandbox and let the kids dig away.
    2. Hide nickels around the party room Easter Egg Hunt style.
    3. Plan a progressive scavenger hunt where the first clue leads to 2nd, and the 2nd leads to 3rd, etc. The final clue guides kids to a hidden treasure chest of pennies or nickels.
- **Target Practice:** Make targets with hung-up hula hoops, plastic cups stacked in the hallway, or poster board with holes cut out. Then, let kids practice their aim. Nerf type arrows or homemade slingshots made with long rubber bands and damp cotton balls are safe options.

- ♥ **Bright Idea!** *There are companies that rent Nerf darts if you go this route and need plenty.*

- ♥ **Bright Idea!** *To avoid chaos, make it clear from the beginning that kids & pets are not targets.*

- • **Movie Time:** As the party winds down, put on the animated *Robin Hood* movie to play in the background. This will help to calm party kids and reduce chaos when it's time to leave.

Invitation

To save you time, we have an invitation on the next page that you may copy and use. Easy peasy!

- ♥ **Bright Idea!** *For some creative fun, use dampened tea bags to give the invitation edges an old-time look.*

NOTES:

____

____

____

____

____

____

____

____

____

ROYAL ARCHERY CONTEST

BY ROYAL DECREE OF NOTTINGHAM CASTLE,
YOUR PRESENCE IS REQUESTED.   BRING
YOUR BEST AIM AND JOIN US IN BIRTHDAY FUN!

HOSTED BY:

AT NOTTINGHAM CASTLE:

DATE:

TIME:

ROYAL RSVP:

Jungle Animal Party

Celebrate friends of the wild and have party kids bring a favorite stuffed animal. It's a perfect theme for boys and girls.

Menu

Make a menu of jungle fare such as nuts, berries and leaves:

- **Jungle Food:** Make homemade trail mix of baked goldfish shaped crackers, sunflower seeds and dried raisins or berries. It's optional to add animal crackers, too.
- **Sliced Grapes with Mint Leaves:** Slice grapes and decorate with mint leaves. Prepare the night before to infuse a little of the mint flavor.
- **Elephant Ear Chips:** Freeze dried apple chips are crunchy, healthy and delicious.
- **Egg Faces:** Make deviled egg faces using pimentos for the eyes and noses.
- **Stuffed Leaves:** Wrap tuna salad in lettuce leaves for fun finger food.
- **Zebra 'Cupcakes':** Try our Pleasing Pumpkin Muffins (recipe on page 97) in place of sugary cupcakes. Use black icing to make zebra stripes on top of each muffin.

- ♥ **Bright Idea!** *It's best to avoid peanuts in party snacks due to possible allergies. To avoid choking hazards, opt for toasted oats for kids under five years old.*
- ♥ **Bright Idea!** *For quick slicing, place grapes in between two plates and carefully run a knife through the middle.*
- ♥ **Bright Idea!** *Make your deviled eggs using light mayonnaise for a healthy bite.*

Decorations

- **Zebra Jungle:** Hang black and white streamers along hallways and the party room wall.
- **Jungle Entrance:** Hang green streamers at the front door like a leafy screen.
- **Jungle Animals:** Decorate the table and food with small plastic animals. Bags of plastic animals can usually be found at a local $1 store.
- **Menu Cards:** Fold index cards in half and write the jungle name of each menu item and place in front of it on the food table.

- ♥ **Bright Idea!** *Add left over plastic jungle animals to party gift bags.*
- ♥ **Bright Idea!** *Add fun jungle animal stickers to the menu cards if you have some on-hand.*

Activities

Keep the kids busy with these:

- **Musical Chairs:** Use stuffed animals to play this classic game by having kids place them in open seats when the music stops. Choose from fun animal songs such as Old McDonald Had a Farm, Bingo, Five Little Monkeys, Itsy Bitsy Spider, Baa Baa Black Sheep or Pop Goes the Weasel.
- **Memory Game:** Use the animal décor for a memory game. Place 5-10 animals on a tray and set it out for kids to view for one minute. Remove the tray and hand kids a pencil and paper. For one minute, have them write down all the animals that they saw on the tray.

- ♥ **Bright Idea!** *For kids who can't write yet, have them draw the animals and add a few minutes to the timer.*

- **Pin the Tail On…:** Grab the classic game at a party store or draw your own jungle animal on poster board. Let the birthday boy or girl choose an animal for this game. Tape is a safer option than actual pins.
- **Animal Hide and Seek:** Gather the stuffed animals that were brought to the party and hide them in a couple of designated rooms. If you don't have a teen or adult helper, then kids can take turns hiding other kids' animals. Once a kid locates her/his own animal, they can help others.

- ♥ **Bright Idea!** *Provide a few extra stuffed animals in case a child is nervous about having her/his furry buddy hidden.*

- **Face Painting/Balloon Animals:** If you're the crafty type or know someone who is, try a little face painting. Or, opt for a pack of specialty balloons and show kids how to make an easy balloon animal. Craft stores have great step-by-step kits for face painting and YouTube has useful videos on how to make balloon animals with kids.
- **Movie Time:** As the party winds down, put on The Jungle Book animated movie or We Bought a Zoo movie to play in the background. This will help to calm party kids and reduce chaos when it's time to leave.

Invitation

To save you time, we have an invitation on the next page that you may copy and use. Easy peasy!

- ♥ **Bright Idea!** *Be sure to ask kids to bring a favorite stuffed animal to the party.*

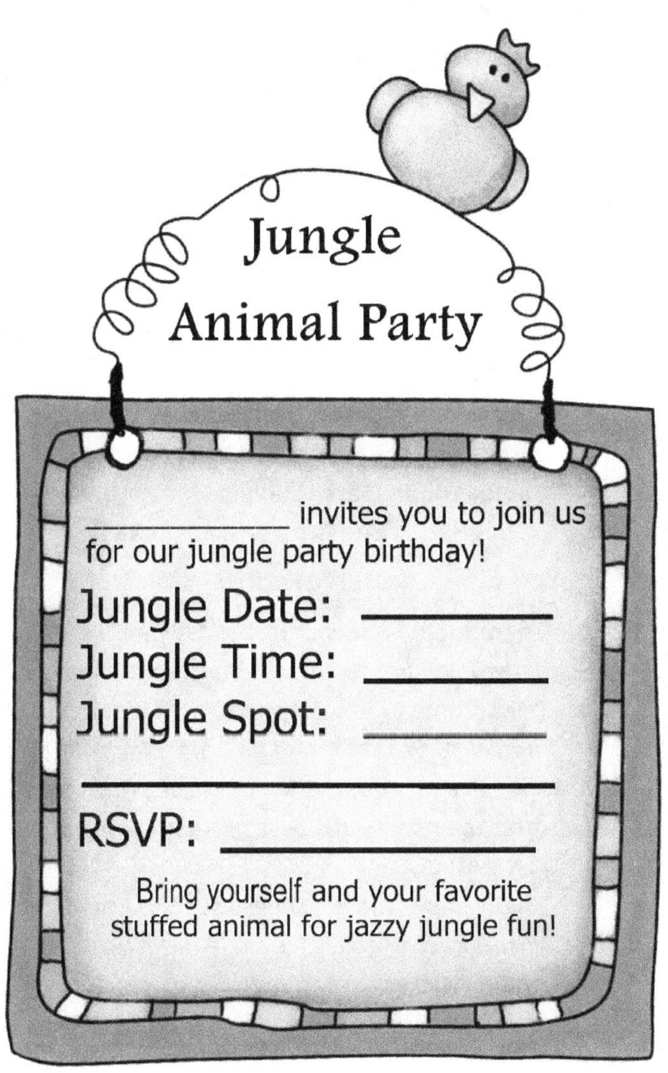
Jungle
Animal Party
_______________ invites you to join us
for our jungle party birthday!
Jungle Date: _______
Jungle Time: _______
Jungle Spot: _______

RSVP: _______________
Bring yourself and your favorite
stuffed animal for jazzy jungle fun!

Classic Games Party

Go a little retro with a classic games party for boys, girls, or both. This is a great time to literally play with food!

Menu

- **Checker Board Fruit Platter:** Place plastic wrap tightly over a regular checker board. Then, arrange sliced kiwi and banana circles like checkers.
- **Pretzel and Olive Tic Tac Toe:** Use thin craft tape to make tic tac toe boards on paper plates.
- **Cheese and Crackers Platter:** Stay with a checkerboard theme with square cheese slices on round crackers.
- **Apple Blondie Bars:** Serve as the party dessert (recipe on page 100). See Activities: Cake Walk.

- ♥ **Bright idea!** *Spritz banana slices with a little orange or pineapple juice to keep them from turning brown.*
- ♥ **Bright Idea!** *Kids can team up to play tic tac toe using pretzel sticks for 'X' and green or black olives for 'O'. If you have an odd number of guests, have an adult join in. After the games, it's best to trash these edible game pieces and snack on the fresh ones.*
- ♥ **Bright Idea!** *Natural cheese such as Muenster, Swiss, Cheddar, or Mozzarella is a healthier choice. Whole wheat crackers are a healthier choice, too.*

Decorations

- **Tic Tac Toe Plates:** Use thin craft tape to make tic tac toe boards on paper plates.
- **Twister Tablecloth:** Use a retro Twister sheet as the party tablecloth. The Twister game can be found at most big-box retailers.

- **Game Bucket Table Centerpiece:** Place a plastic bucket
  in the center of the table filled with fun game goodies.
  Rubik's cubes, decks of cards, dice, dominoes, jump
  ropes, jacks and Yahtzee are fun for multiple age groups
  of girls or boys. Jump ropes and cards make great party
  gifts, too.

Activities

Keep the kids busy with these:

- **Cake Walk:**
    1. Write a number on 8 ½ x 11 inch pieces of
       construction paper or newspaper - one for each
       child at the party. Lay out pieces of paper in a
       wide circle on the floor.
    2. Play music while kids walk in a circle stepping
       on the numbered sheets.
    3. When the music stops, have all kids freeze,
       trying to step on the closest number.
    4. Draw a number – same as numbers on the
       pieces of paper on floor – that parent keeps
       track of in a bag.
    5. Announce the number, see which child is
       stepping on the number & make them winner
       of that round of the game.
    6. Give the round winner an Apple Blondie dessert
       bar and have them sit at the eating table.
    7. Remove winning number paper from the game
       circle.
    8. Start music again.
    9. Repeat process until all party kids are sitting
       and enjoying an Apple Blondie dessert bar.

- **Simon Says:**
    1. Designate one person as Simon who announces to the group of kids silly things to do. For example, if he/she announces, "Simon says, touch your nose," then all kids must touch their nose. Or, for example, if he/she announces simply, "Touch your nose," then all kids must do nothing.
    2. Have 'Simon' continue to give the group of kids commands, by starting with 'Simon says' or not.
    3. When kids forget to follow what 'Simon Says' or not, then they sit down.
    4. Repeat process of 'Simon says' or not, until only one child is standing.
    5. The winner is last child standing.

♥ **Bright Idea!** *Have 'Simon' wear a silly hat with a big 'S' on it. Find a hat around the house and use a rubber-banded piece of paper with 'S' or a fabric 'S' on it.*

- **Red Light, Green Light:**
    1. Designate one child to be the Stoplight. This child must look to the front of the room so she/he cannot see the other kids behind her/him.
    2. Line up all other party kids about 15 feet behind the Stoplight, looking to the front of the room.
    3. Have the Stoplight announce "green light" or "red light."
    4. When Stoplight announces "green light" then all kids may slowly take baby steps toward Stoplight.
    5. When Stoplight announces "red light" then all kids must freeze.

6. Stoplight turns toward the other kids on 'red light' to see if they catch anyone moving. Anyone caught moving on a 'red light' must sit down.
7. Repeat process of 'red light' or 'green light' until one child sneaks up and touches Stoplight.
8. The sneaky child is winner.

♥ **Bright Idea!** *Ask the birthday boy or girl if they want to be Stoplight first? Or, if not, have him/her choose the Stoplight.*

- **Rotate Game Stations:** If party kids are old enough to play games on their own, set up a few game stations and break the kids into groups rotating every 20 minutes. Some games that can be played in 20 minutes are Checkers, Dominoes, War – with a deck of cards, Puzzles, and dress up like a clown/princess/pirate/etc.]

- **Movie Time:** As the party winds down, put on *Candyland: The Great Lollipop Adventure, Charlie and the Chocolate Factory* or *Mary Poppins* to play in the background. This will help to calm party kids and reduce the chaos when it's time to leave.

Invitation

To save you time, we have an invitation on the next page that you may copy and use. Easy peasy!

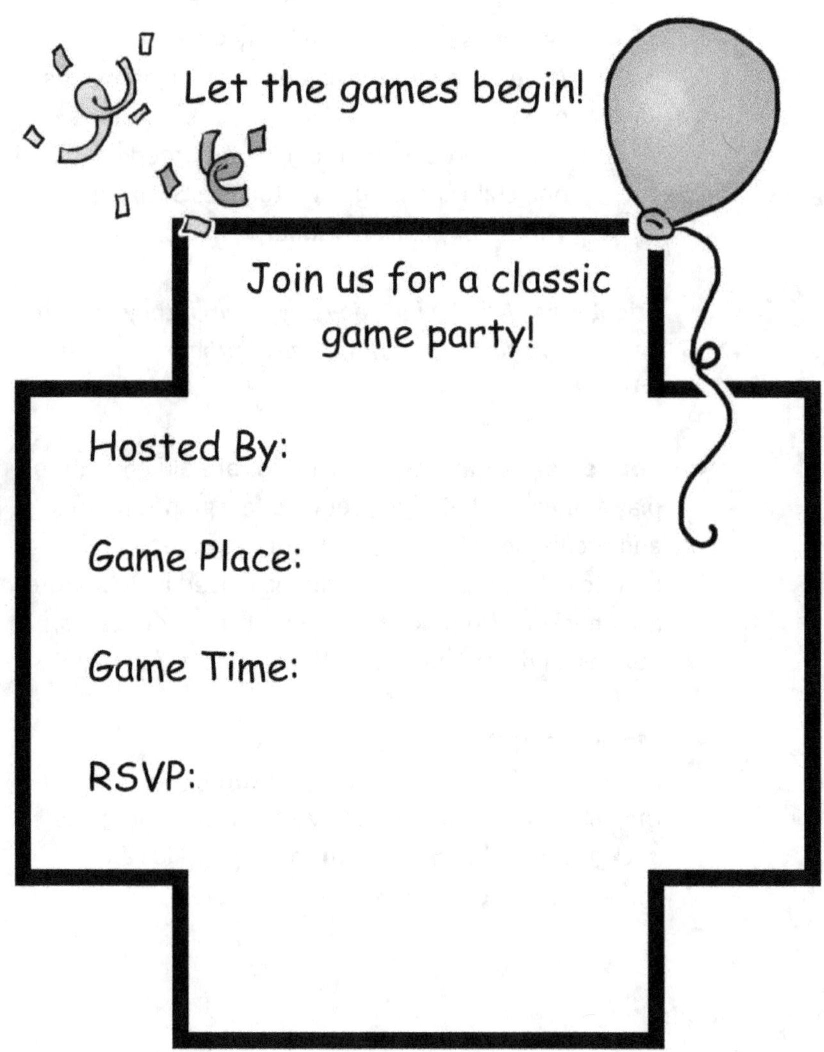

Let the games begin!

Join us for a classic
game party!

Hosted By:

Game Place:

Game Time:

RSVP:

5 Slow Cooker Recipes

These recipes literally cook themselves after a bit of morning prep. Take care of everything else in your busy day and come home to a homemade dinner.

Barley, Mushroom and Chickpea Soup

- Servings: 6-8
- Cooking time: 7-8 hours, low

1 tablespoon **Olive oil**, extra virgin
16 ounces **Mushrooms**, sliced
1 medium **Onion**, chopped
3-4 cloves **Garlic**, minced
4 cups **Vegetable broth**
1 cup **Water**
2 tablespoons **Tomato paste**
1 can, 15 ounces **Chickpeas**, drained
1 cup **Carrots**, peeled and cut into matchsticks or coins
1 cup **Celery**, chopped
½ teaspoon each **Dried oregano** and **basil leaves**
1 teaspoon **Dried thyme leaves**
1/3 cup **Barley**, pearled - not quick cooking kind
½ cup Fresh **parsley**, chopped
Pinch **Salt** and **Black pepper**

1. Get out a large skillet and heat the olive oil over medium heat. Add mushrooms, onions, garlic and stir until vegetables are golden.
2. Add the mushroom mixture into a slow cooker along with broth, tomato paste, chickpeas, carrots, celery, oregano, basil, thyme, barley, salt and black pepper.
3. Cover and cook on low for 7-8 hours.
4. Add chopped parsley in the last 15 minutes of cooking.
5. Add a garnish of chopped parsley on each soup bowl.
6. Serve with whole grain crackers & cheese, and fresh fruit for dessert.

Orange Asian Chicken
- Servings: 4
- Cooking time: 4 hours, low

2 pounds **Chicken thighs**, boneless and skinless (or can use breasts)
¼ cup **Orange marmalade/jam**
1 medium **Orange**, zest and juice
¼ cup **Flour**
2 tablespoons **Tomato paste**
¼ cup **Soy sauce**
1 teaspoon **Sesame oil**
1 teaspoon **Garlic powder**
½ tablespoon **Spicy spice rub**, any flavor

1. Spray the inside of slow cooker with vegetable oil spray.
2. Add ingredients into the slow cooker.
3. Stir well.
4. Cover and cook on low for 4 hours.
5. Stir halfway through if you are home.
6. Serve with steamed brown rice or whole wheat pasta & broccoli.

Island Coconut Pork Stew

- Servings: 6
- Cooking time: 6 hours, low

1 tablespoon **Olive oil**, extra virgin
2 pounds **Pork tenderloin**, cut into 2 inch chunks
¼ teaspoon each **Salt** and **Black pepper**
1 large **Onion**, sliced thinly
1 large **Green Bell pepper**, seeds removed and sliced thinly
1-1/2 cups **Baby carrots**
1 can, 14 ounces **Coconut milk**, light
2 tablespoons **Curry powder**
1 tablespoon **Soy sauce**
½ teaspoon **Ground ginger**
1 teaspoon **Garlic powder**
¼-1/2 teaspoon **Crushed red pepper flakes**
1 cup **Plain yogurt**, low fat, for garnish
½ cup Fresh **cilantro** or **parsley**, for garnish

1. Get out a large skillet and heat the olive oil over medium heat. Add chunks of pork, sprinkle with salt and pepper, and sear them by getting all sides to contact the pan, about 3-4 minutes. Do not cook pork, just sear the outside.
2. In a bowl, mix together all other ingredients except yogurt and fresh parsley/cilantro garnishes.
3. Add seared pork and mixed sauce into the slow cooker.
4. Stir well.
5. Cover and cook on low for 6 hours.
6. Stir halfway through if you are home.
7. Serve with plain yogurt and fresh parsley or cilantro as garnishes. Soft pita or flat bread may also be served on the side along with cut-up mango for dessert.

Easy Beef Stew

- Servings: 6
- Cooking time: 8 hours, low

2 pounds **Beef round roast**, or, beef sirloin roast, cut into 1 ½-inch chunks
¼ cup **Flour**
2 cans, 14 ounces **Diced tomatoes with green chilies**
½ cup **Water**
1/8 teaspoon **Salt** & **pepper**
10 small **Potatoes**, white or red skinned, with skin left on, cut in half
½ pound **Baby carrots**, whole

1. Add all ingredients into the slow cooker.
2. Stir well.
3. Cover and cook on low for 8 hours.
4. Stir halfway through if you are home.
5. Serve with a leafy green salad and sliced apples for dessert.

Note: The tomatoes with chilies add some spicy heat to this stew. If you prefer it to be less spicy then feel free to substitute one or both cans of tomatoes with plain diced tomatoes.

Magical Turkey Breast

- Servings: 8-12
- Cooking time: 8 hours, low

1 Frozen Turkey Breast

1. Add frozen (not thawed) turkey breast small enough to fit into the slow cooker, meaty side up.
2. Cover and cook on low for 8 hours.
3. Serve as a hot turkey sandwich with gravy and cranberry sauce, or serve as sliced turkey with a baked sweet potato and steamed green beans.

Note: Feel free to sprinkle the frozen turkey breast with dry herbs and or spices before starting to cook. However, you do not need to add anything to the slow cooker along with the turkey.

More Recipes

These recipes are everyday winners that can be made by anyone in the family. If your kids are school-aged, then get them to help with supervision.

Broccoli with Cheese
Here's a broccoli recipe the whole family will love!
Kids can help by measuring the ingredients and sprinkling the cheese, with supervision.

Makes 6 servings

4 cups **Broccoli**
1 cup **Cheddar cheese**, natural, shredded or grated
1 tsp **Paprika** (optional, adds natural color)

1. Wash broccoli well in cool tap water. Shake off extra water.
2. Trim any dry ends from broccoli stalk.
3. Cut entire broccoli bunch into bite-size pieces.
4. Place into a microwave-safe dish and add about ½ inch water.
5. Cover dish with microwavable lid or waxed paper.
6. Cook on high until tender-crisp, about 5-7 minutes depending on power of oven.
7. Drain water and place broccoli into a serving bowl.
8. Sprinkle with cheese and paprika.

Pleasing Pumpkin Muffins

Create these muffins for hungry and healthy kids!

Kids can help by cracking the eggs, measuring the ingredients, stirring the batter and filling the muffin pans, with supervision.

Makes 12 regular or about 24 mini muffins

1 can, 15-16 oz **Pumpkin**, solid pack, canned
½ cup **Sugar**
2 **Eggs**, large
2 Tbsp **Unsweetened applesauce**
2 Tbsp **Canola** <u>or</u> light-flavored olive oil
½ cup **Water**
¾ cup **White flour**
¾ cup **Whole wheat flour**
½ tsp **Baking soda**
¾ tsp **Baking powder**
¼ tsp **Salt**
1 tsp **Pumpkin pie spice** <u>or</u> ½ tsp each, cinnamon and nutmeg
1 cup **Raisins**, optional

1. Preheat oven to 400 degrees.
2. Get out a large bowl and add the wet ingredients: pumpkin, sugar, eggs, applesauce, oil and water.
3. With an electric mixer or hand whisk, mix up everything for 1-2 minutes.
4. In a different bowl, add the dry ingredients: white flour, whole wheat flour, baking soda, baking powder, salt, spice and raisins. Stir up with a spoon until well mixed.
5. Add the dry ingredients to the wet ingredients slowly. Mix with an electric mixer or a big, wooden spoon until everything is moist. Do not over mix.
6. Lightly spray the muffin pan(s) with vegetable oil cooking spray.
7. Using a soup spoon, fill the muffin pans about halfway full.
8. Place into the oven and bake for 20 minutes.

Chocolate-y Banana Cupcakes

This kid-pleasing dessert is so good, you can skip the icing!

Kids can help by measuring the ingredients, cracking the egg, mashing the banana, stirring the batter and filling the cupcake pans, with supervision.

Makes 12 regular or about 24 mini muffins

½ cup **Sugar**
1/2 cup **White flour**
1/2 cup **Whole wheat flour**
½ cup **Cocoa powder**, unsweetened version with single ingredient—just cocoa
¾ teaspoon **Baking powder**
¾ teaspoon **Baking soda**
¼ teaspoon **Salt** (optional)
1 **Egg**, large
1 **Banana**, large, ripe, mashed
½ cup **Water**
¼ cup **Milk, 1%**
3 tablespoons **Canola** or light flavored olive oil
1 teaspoon **Vanilla extract**

1. Preheat oven to 350 degrees.
2. Line cupcake (muffin) pans with paper liners or spray lightly with vegetable oil spray – to prevent sticking to pan.
3. Mix together these dry ingredients in a large bowl: sugar, flours, cocoa powder, baking powder, baking soda and salt. Set aside.
4. Mix together these wet ingredients in a medium bowl: egg, mashed banana, water, milk, oil, vanilla extract.
5. Add the wet ingredients to the dry ingredients, then stir to combine. Stir just until mixed together.
6. Using a soup spoon or liquid measuring cup, fill cupcake pans about half to 2/3 full.
7. Go back and add a little to each cupcake if you need to use up the batter. Batter will expand in the oven as it cooks.

8. Place cupcake pans into the oven and bake for 20 minutes.
9. Test for doneness by inserting a toothpick into the center of the cupcake. If the toothpick comes out clean, then the cupcake is done. If not, place pan back into the oven for 2-3 minutes and test again.

Bunny Rabbit Salad

Here's a recipe that works as a side dish any day of the week! Kids can help by measuring the ingredients, grating the carrots and stirring everything up, with supervision.

Makes 6 servings

3 large **Carrots**
1 cup **Pineapple** tidbits or crushed, canned and drained well
1 cup **Yogurt**, plain, nonfat
½ teaspoon **Vanilla extract**
½ tablespoon **Sugar**

1. Peel carrots and remove both ends.
2. Rinse carrots in cool tap water and pat dry.
3. Grate carrots with a hand grater or food processor.
4. Place carrots and drained pineapple into a medium sized bowl.
5. In a separate small bowl, make a creamy sauce by mixing up the yogurt, vanilla and sugar with a spoon.
6. Add sauce to carrots-pineapple and stir everything together.

Apple Blondie Bars
Here's a fruit-y twist on a simple butterscotch blondie, with less sugar too!

Kids can help by measuring the ingredients, cracking the eggs, picking out the apple, stirring the batter and spooning the batter into the pan, with supervision.

Makes 24-28 bars

1-1/2 cups **White flour**
1/2 cup **Whole wheat flour**
2 teaspoons **Baking powder**
Pinch **Salt**
½-1 teaspoon **Cinnamon**
½ cup **Butter**, softened (not melted)
1 cup **Brown sugar**, not packed down
2 large **Eggs**
1 teaspoon **Vanilla**
1 medium **Apple**, any variety, skin-on, chopped
1 cup **Raisins** or **Walnuts**, optional

1. Preheat the oven to 350 degrees.
2. In a medium bowl, measure and stir up the flours, baking powder, salt, and cinnamon. Set this aside.
3. In a large mixing bowl, measure and add the butter, brown sugar, eggs, and vanilla. Mix this with an electric mixer or stir with a wooden spoon until it is smooth.
4. Add the wet ingredients into the dry mixed ingredients. Stir.
5. Add chopped apple. Add the raisins and/or walnuts. Stir briefly, just to mix. Try not to over-mix the batter.
6. Spray 13 x 9 inch baking pan with vegetable oil spray.

7. Spoon batter into the pan and smooth out the top with a knife or spatula.

8. Bake for 30-35 minutes. Test doneness at 30 minutes by inserting a table knife into middle of the cooked bars. If it comes out clean, they are done. If not, put back into the oven for 3-5 minutes and re-test.

Roasted Vegetables

Roasting vegetables sweetens up their flavors for kids of all ages.

Makes 4-6 servings

4-5 cups **Vegetables**, cut into 1 inch bite size pieces (try broccoli, sweet Bell peppers, sweet or white potatoes, carrots, green beans, asparagus and turnips)
1 tablespoon **Extra virgin olive oil**
Pinch **Salt**, **pepper** and/or **dried herbs**

1. Preheat oven to 425 degrees F.
2. Wash veggies with cool water in the kitchen sink.
3. Cut veggies, if needed, into bite-size pieces (about 1 inch x 1 inch)
4. Place veggies into a large bowl and drizzle them with a small amount of extra virgin olive oil. For example, 1-2 tablespoons for a full sheet pan of veggies; ½-1 tablespoon for half a sheet pan of veggies.
5. Scatter veggies onto a sheet pan, in a single layer, and dust lightly with salt, pepper and/or dried herbs you like.
6. Put pan into preheated oven for 20-25 minutes.
7. Test doneness by poking with a fork. They should be tender but not mushy.

Fresh Apple Salad
This is a 'go to' side dish for any meal!
Kids can help by washing the apples, squeezing the lemon,
stirring and sprinkling the salad, with supervision.

Makes 4 servings

3 medium **Apples**, any kind, any color
1 teaspoon **Lemon juice**, squeezed from a fresh lemon
3/4 cup, 5-6 ounces **Lemon or lime yogurt**, made from nonfat milk
¼ cup **Plain yogurt**, made from nonfat milk
¼ teaspoon **Ground cinnamon**

1. Wash apples and pat dry with a clean towel.
2. Cut apples in half. Cut in half again.
3. Remove core and seeds from apples.
4. Cut apples into bite-size pieces and place into a medium or large bowl.
5. Squeeze lemon juice all over the apple pieces. Stir up with a big spoon.
6. Measure and add yogurt (both kinds) to the apples. Stir gently.
7. Sprinkle cinnamon over the top of the salad.

Easy Pumpkin Pie

This pie is made in the blender so it's super quick and easy! Kids can help by measuring the ingredients and loading them into the blender, with supervision.

Makes 8 servings

1 can, 15-16 ounces **Pumpkin**, solid pack
1 can, 12 ounces **Evaporated skim milk**
2 large **Eggs**
½ cup **Sugar**
½ cup **Baking Mix**, Heart Healthy kind
2 teaspoons **Pumpkin pie spice**
2 teaspoons **Vanilla extract**

1. Preheat oven to 350 degrees.
2. Measure all ingredients into a blender.
3. Blend on low to medium speed about 1-2 minutes, until smooth.
4. Pour pumpkin filling into a pie pan that is lightly sprayed with oil.
5. Bake pie in the oven for 50-55 minutes.
6. Pie is done when a small knife poked into the center comes out clean.
7. Cool the pie for 20-30 minutes before eating. May cover and store in fridge up to 3 days.

About Cindy

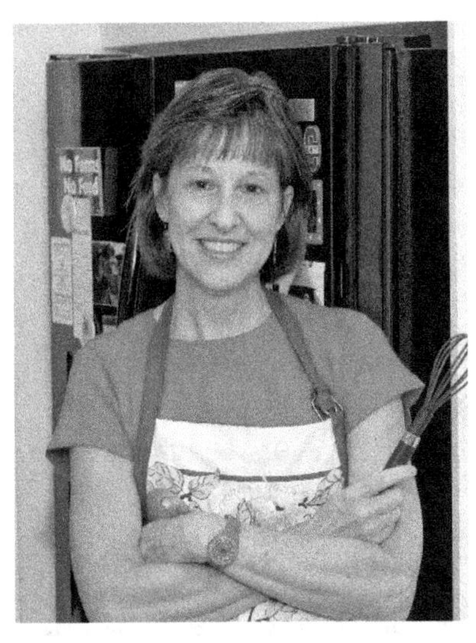

Growing up in an active family where simple, balanced meals were the norm, Cindy learned early on about good nutrition. It was no coincidence that she chose to pursue a science major in college and, later, a master's degree in food science and nutrition along with her RDN, registered dietitian nutritionist, credential. Cindy has enjoyed the variety of her career. Since 2010, she has owned and operated Market Basket Nutrition (marketbasketnutrition.com), her nutrition education and counseling business based in Winston-Salem, NC. In her practice, Cindy helps busy people learn skills in tasty meal planning, smarter grocery shopping, and preparing home-based meals with simple and nutritious ingredients. She has fun testing recipes on her son and husband and Cindy relaxes by walking, swimming, gardening and listening to all kinds of music.

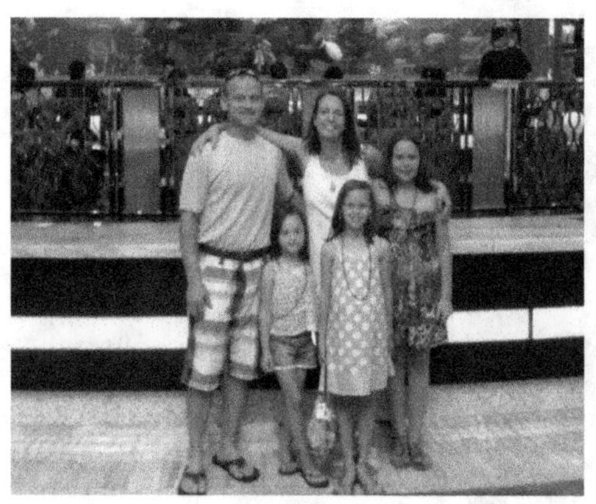

About Andrea

A mother of three, Andrea has been managing her family and freelance writing for twenty plus years. Her creative plate is eclectic including screenplays, magazine articles, book reviews and video editing. She enjoys the challenge of making dinnertime fun and is currently working on a theme dinner book with the guidance of her children and husband who is a high school teacher.

When she isn't working, she enjoys exploring our beautiful country with her family which has included a cross country trek from North Carolina to California and back, a road trip to the Mall of America and an amusement park themed trip through the northeastern US. Next on the list, is a cross country journey to the Pacific Northwest which is set to include overnighting in a treehouse.

www.ingramcontent.com/pod-product-compliance
Lightning Source LLC
Chambersburg PA
CBHW051755250726
48659CB00001B/427